# The Cholesterol Myth
Lower Cholesterol Won't Stop Heart Disease Only
Healthy Cholesterol Will

*Use This Cholesterol Recipe Book and Cholesterol Diet
To Lower Cholesterol Naturally Keep Cholesterol
Healthy And Prevent Heart Disease.*

By John McArthur and Cheri Merz

# Copyright

All rights reserved worldwide. No part of this publication may be replicated, redistributed, or given away in any form without the prior written consent of the author/publisher or the terms relayed to you herein.

**Natural Health Magazine**

**www.naturalhealthmagazine.net**

The information in this book is provided for educational and information purposes only. It is not intended to be used as medical advice or as a substitute for treatment by a doctor or healthcare provider.

The information and opinions contained in this publication are believed to be accurate based on the information available to the author. However, the contents have not been evaluated by the U.S. Food and Drug Administration and are not intended to diagnose, treat, cure or prevent disease.

The author and publisher are not responsible for the use, effectiveness or safety of any procedure or treatment mentioned in this book. The publisher is not responsible for errors and omissions.

**Warning**

All treatment of any medical condition (without exception) must always be done under supervision of a qualified medical professional. The fact that a substance is "natural" does not necessarily mean that it has no side effects or interaction with other medications.

Medical professionals are qualified and experienced to give advice on side effects and interactions of all types of medication.

# Table of Contents

Copyright 2

Foreword 17

Cholesterol: Is It Really the Villain? 19

What is cholesterol and what role does it play in our bodies? 21

Cholesterol Myths 25

Cholesterol and Genes 29

Honing in on the real villain - oxidized cholesterol 32

The Anti-Inflammation Diet 49

Dr. Weil's Anti-Inflammatory Pyramid 62

Your Healthy Cholesterol Shopping List 70

Part 2 - Recipes To Keep Your Cholesterol Healthy 75

Chicken Recipes 75

Fish Recipes 105

Beef and Veal Recipes 149

Lamb Recipes 163

Pork Recipes 174

Salad Recipes 189

Vegetable Dishes 249

Soup Recipes 316

Muesli, Nuts and Fruit Recipes 322

Smoothie Recipes 347

Bibliography 366

**More Books by John McArthur 366**

# Foreword

What you are about to learn may shock you!

- There is no such thing as 'good' cholesterol or 'bad' cholesterol. All cholesterol plays an important part in your body's healthy functioning.
- 95% of the cholesterol circulating in your blood stream is made by your body—not from dietary cholesterol.
- The western medical establishment, aided and abetted by the FDA, has used bad science and faulty reasoning to frighten an unsuspecting public into taking billions of dollars' worth of cholesterol and heart medications that are questionable at best, and yet we are actually less healthy as a nation than we were before any of these medications were created.
- Few doctors will admit what the real culprit is, or teach you to cure it.
- It is easy to make the lifestyle changes that will avoid, perhaps even cure, atherosclerosis, 'high cholesterol' and heart disease without medication, without surgery and without depriving you of delicious foods you can eat in plenty.
- The best way to improve your cholesterol is to get half an hour of aerobic exercise per day and to lose weight, which

you can do easily by incorporating exercise and healthy food choices.

# Cholesterol: Is It Really the Villain?

No doubt the word cholesterol summons the image in your mind of clogged arteries, fatty foods, and perhaps your doctor warning you that if you don't get yours under control, you will have a heart attack, or at the very least have to take medication for the rest of your life. You have seen countless ads on TV warning of the dangers of cholesterol, and may have read articles about so-called 'good' cholesterol and 'bad' cholesterol, as if some cholesterol—the bad kind—were an out-of-control animal that might attack you. It is time to dispel the myths and inexact science that shock journalism has planted in your mind and learn to take control of your health the natural way. In truth, there is no such thing as 'good' cholesterol or 'bad' cholesterol. All cholesterol types play an essential role in the body, which is why most of the serum cholesterol circulating in your blood is manufactured by your own body.

If someone asked you where most of the cholesterol in your body comes from you might say, "Well, of course it comes from the foods I eat!" You may be surprised to know that as much as 95% of the cholesterol in your body is in fact manufactured by your own liver. Your liver works diligently to produce 3000 milligrams of cholesterol daily, which constitutes the majority of the cholesterol in your body. Only 5% of it comes from the foods you eat. The question you may be asking now is why would our bodies be manufacturing so much of something that is the cause of so many life-threatening health issues? It may surprise you to know that your fear of eggs and other cholesterol-rich foods came from an inaccurate understanding on the part of conventional medical researchers decades ago.

The fact is that your body actually needs a certain amount of cholesterol to function properly – so much so that your liver supplies most of it by itself. Our bodies use cholesterol to produce Vitamin D and certain hormones and it plays a vital role in the repairing of damaged cells. Cholesterol is also instrumental in the production of bile, which is an important stomach acid used by your body during digestion and in the prevention of a build-up of cholesterol in your blood stream. What you don't know about cholesterol can and will hurt you.

As you can see, cholesterol in and of itself is not bad at all. The fact is that it is essential to your health, but can be harmful under certain circumstances. That is why it is crucial to know the facts. Having misconceptions about the causes of high cholesterol, what your doctor even means by high cholesterol, and harboring erroneous ideas surrounding methods of managing blood cholesterol levels can be harmful in the long run. Have you considered that you have not been informed of the newer research because it would hurt sales of cholesterol-lowering medicine? Yes, that is a strong accusation. But consider this: who has the monetary upper hand, the various cooperative marketing organizations that egg farmers and beef ranchers rely upon to get their message out, or drug manufacturers who constantly lobby doctors to prescribe their drugs and bombard you with frightening TV ads? And which sells more newspapers and magazines, good news or bad? In fact, the truth is out there, but you must dig to find it. Alternatively, read on for a full discussion of what cholesterol is and is not — that is, not the villain. □

## What is cholesterol and what role does it play in our bodies?

According to the National Institutes of Health website, *"Cholesterol is an unsaturated alcohol of the steroid family of compounds; it is essential for the normal function of all animal cells and is a fundamental element of their cell membranes. It is also a precursor of various critical substances such as adrenal and gonadal steroid hormones and bile acids. Triglycerides are fatty acid esters of glycerol and represent the main lipid component of dietary fat and fat deposits of animals."*

Cholesterol is usually described as a soft, waxy material found among the fats (also known as lipids) in the bloodstream and it is a vital part necessary for the maintenance of all our body's cells. It plays a critical role in the manufacture of important male and female sex hormones and steroidal hormones, including pregnenolone, testosterone, estrogen, progesterone, and cortisol. Those hormones are essential for the health of the immune system, the mineral-regulating functions of the kidneys, and the smooth running of the hormonal systems in men and women.

Cholesterol and triglycerides are insoluble in water, and therefore must be transported within the plasma associated with various lipoproteins, the cholesterol portion being the 'lipo-' or fat part of the molecule, and the protein carrying it being the rest of the molecule. There are five major classes of these lipoproteins, classed by hydrated density, electrophoretic mobility (how fast they travel under certain study conditions), size, and relative ratios of cholesterol, triglycerides and proteins. Those classes are known as chylomicrons, very-low-density lipoproteins (VLDL), intermediate-density lipoproteins (IDL), low-density lipoproteins (LDL), and high-density lipoproteins (HDL). The roles of each of these substances in your body and how damage to them can harm you, will be discussed as we go forward. We will primarily be concerned with three of them: VLDL, LDL and HDL. For now, suffice it to say that VLDL and LDL are tasked with carrying cholesterol that is needed by your cells from the liver to their destination. HDL is the return process, whereby cholesterol is returned to the liver to be broken down and then either recycled or expelled from your body.

As a review, there are several main functions of cholesterol in your body, each as vital to your health and well-being as any other substance your glands manufacture. They are:

- It plays an important role in the build up and maintenance of the body's cells.
- It is involved in the determining which molecules are allowed to pass into cells and which cannot (cell membrane permeability)
- It assists the body in the productions of sex hormones (testosterone and estrogens)
- It assists the body in the production of hormones released by the adrenal glands (cortisol, corticosterone, aldosterone, and others)
- It assists the body in the production of bile
- It is involved in the synthesis of Vitamin D, deficiency of which is implicated in heart disease and impaired immune function
- It plays a crucial role in the metabolism of vitamins E, A, D and K, all of which are fat soluble.
- It helps nerve signals travel they way they should by insulating nerve fibers.

LDL has erroneously been characterized as 'bad' cholesterol, for reasons we will explore later, and by the same token HDL has been characterized as good. As we will see, these characterizations are overly general, based on a poor understanding of what roles cholesterol plays in the body, not especially accurate with regard to previous medical research into the causes of lifestyle diseases, and not helpful in protecting your own health. That is not to say that cholesterol has not been implicated in plaque formation and coronary heart disease; it has. However, current research shows that elevated levels of serum cholesterol are not the only cause, nor necessarily the cause at all, of these ailments. In fact, the disease process is much more complex than can be explained simply by elevated cholesterol levels.

It is a fact of Western medicine that we usually identify and treat illnesses in isolation from the whole body, seeing it as a sort of mechanical device that can be kept running by repairing or replacing any malfunctioning parts, as long as it doesn't blow up before we get to the repair. Alternative medicine and holistic approaches are often maligned as inferior; but what is really inferior? Is it medicine that takes into account the fact that all our physical processes are interlinked, or is it the 'repair or replace' mentality that sees heart disease as separate from endocrine disease, arthritis and other autoimmune diseases; as primary rather than symptomatic of something else that has gone wrong with our machine? If you were to undertake a study of common illnesses that are epidemic in today's world, you would soon begin to detect a pattern and relationships between the breakdown of the core internal processes that are designed to keep us healthy and any number of seemingly unrelated illnesses that conventional medical doctors treat in isolation. Heart disease is a case in point. Later we will explore the cause of the breakdown, but first, how did high cholesterol come to be associated with heart disease?

# Cholesterol Myths

In his excellent book "The Great Cholesterol Lie: Why Inflammation Kills and the Real Cure for Heart Disease" Dr. Dwight Lundell states:

*"All the research into the biological side of heart disease blamed cholesterol as the primary cause of heart disease yet I could never fully connect with that theory. I held this epidemic in my hands, performed 5,000 open heart surgeries battling the epidemic for a quarter of a century. What I saw in surgery contradicted all the data backing the cholesterol theory.*

*Clearly one-half of my heart attack patients had normal cholesterol. When they returned ten years later for a second operation, half still had normal cholesterol levels. Even the nutritional studies didn't show a benefit of a low-fat, low-cholesterol diet so there had to be something else. Something was missing.*

*As the medical community and brilliant physicians continued to believe and endorse the theory, millions of Americans bought into bad advice while statistics grew worse at a terrifying, epidemic rate – the largest in history. I was performing by-pass like it was standard practice bandaging the epidemic. We were mastering the art of saving lives but the numbers kept increasing."*

*emphasis ours

Whether you blame bad science or a pharmaceuticals industry that has a vested interest in selling cholesterol-lowering drugs, it is clear that we have for too long bought into a theory that does not work. How this happened is rather interesting. Dr. Lundell traces a history of the theory, which begins with a high incidence (77%) of soldiers killed during the Korean conflict showing evidence of coronary artery disease at an average age of 22. Naturally, this alarmed the medical establishment and in turn the general public, which demanded answers. If heart disease could strike anyone at any age, what could we do to protect ourselves?

Turning to a long-running study of heart disease, The Framingham Study, a longitudinal project of the National Heart, Lung and Blood Institute and Boston University that is still running today, medical researchers eager for a quick answer to public panic seized upon the statistical fact that approximately half of the study participants had both high cholesterol and heart disease. We should note here that the Framingham Study was and is an observational study. That means that rather than testing a theory against a statistical norm (a control group), or testing two theories against each other, the Framingham Study was designed to gather information over a long period so that statistical conclusions could be reached. It is now into the third generation of participants. The trouble with statistics is that they are sometimes used to bolster weak arguments and can be manipulated to make an unsupported theory appear to be ironclad truth. You may have heard the quote that illustrates this, sometimes attributed to Mark Twain, "There are three kinds of lies; lies, damn lies, and statistics." It is telling that the risk factors now used by doctors to determine whether they should prescribe cholesterol-lowering medications rather than manage high cholesterol via life-style changes is based on the Framingham Study.

Although the study had also identified other risk factors for heart disease, such as smoking, the cholesterol link became the major but narrow focus of the medical establishment from that day forward. That leap was a little like saying 'everyone in this room is a genius; half the people in this room eat salmon; therefore everyone who eats salmon is a genius.' There are two things wrong with this faulty syllogism, as any philosopher would be able to tell you. In the first place, the conclusion is not supported by the premises, much less are the premises valid for the rest of the population not included in the room, or in the case of the Framingham Study, the rest of the world. However, scientists looking for more evidence to fit the theory designed studies that inevitably supported it — another faulty piece of logic that defies the rules of scientific investigation.

A scientist by the name of Ancel Keys (famous for popularizing the Mediterranean diet) conducted a study on the relationship between dietary consumption of fatty foods and heart disease in diverse populations. In 1961, when Dr. Keys was featured on the cover of Time Magazine, his study made a lot of sense. However, the results of the dietary shift that ensued showed that the premise was very wrong. Dr. Lundell states, *"Consumption of dietary fat decreased from the 1960's to the 1990's but the rate of heart disease did not and instead, the incidence of obesity and Type II diabetes soared."*

Politics, scientific studies driven by low budgets rather than good science, and media attention continued to solidify the notion in our collective consciousness that consumption of dietary fat equaled high cholesterol equaled prevalence of heart disease. Dr. Lundell's book reveals a fascinating story of how this myth was conceived, supported and perpetuated to this day, creating a wildly profitable industry for drug manufacturers and pitting the various food industry factions against each other for government support or condemnation of their products. Even our revered food pyramid turns out to have been a creation of the political machine! Meanwhile, study after study failed to prove the association between dietary fat intake and coronary disease and the results were systematically ignored. Again quoting Dr. Lundell:

*After 49 years of research, this means there is no association between the amount of fat in the diet and heart disease. The MRFIT Study, The Physicians Health Study and The Women's Health Initiative Study provide more examples of studies with disappointing results in proving fat and cholesterol theory. These studies showed:*

- *Reducing intake of cholesterol has no effect on the risk of chronic heart disease.*

- *Low-fat diets do not reduce the risk of chronic heart disease.*

- *A daily dose of aspirin (anti-inflammatory) does\* reduce the risk of chronic heart disease.*

*The amazing thing about the studies is they missed the real value of their results. These studies proved what they were expecting to happen did not happen and that something else must be the cause of heart disease.*
\*emphasis ours

Before we talk about what that something else is, we need to explore the role that genetics plays in serum cholesterol levels.

# Cholesterol and Genes

Higher than optimal levels of cholesterol circulating in the blood can be caused by diet, lifestyle factors and even stress; in fact, these are the most prevalent causes. However, about 1 person in 500 have high cholesterol levels (hypercholesterolemia) due to inherited tendencies. Certain populations, including Afrikaners in South Africa, French Canadians, Lebanese, and Finns, see a more frequent occurrence of familial hypercholesterolemia, the most common type of inherited high cholesterol.

Familial hypercholesterolemia is caused by a mutation in one of several genes that provide the instructions your body uses to make a protein called a low-density lipoprotein receptor. This type of receptor binds to the LDL particles which you will recall are the primary carriers of cholesterol in the blood. These receptors play a critical role in regulating cholesterol levels by removing low-density lipoproteins from the bloodstream some of the genetic mutations reduce the number of low-density lipoprotein receptors produced within cells. Others disrupt the receptors' ability to remove low-density lipoproteins from the bloodstream. As a result, people with these mutations have high levels of blood cholesterol, which is deposited in tissues such as the skin, tendons, and arteries that supply blood to the heart as it circulates in the bloodstream.

Another type of inherited hypercholesterolemia is called familial combined hyperlipidemia. This condition is characterized by a high level of fat particles in the blood, including cholesterol. What you should know about it is that it is hereditary and causes high cholesterol as well as high triglycerides, both of which are major risk factors for heart disease under the right circumstances. About 20 percent of the 13 million people in the US who have coronary artery disease and are under age 60 have familial combined hyperlipidemia. It is implicated in heart attacks in younger people, whose high cholesterol can become an issue as early as the teen years, and is more common in families with a history of high cholesterol.

Both of these conditions should be suspected if family history shows a tendency and can be diagnosed both by family history and blood tests that measure serum cholesterol and triglyceride levels. Although genetics does play a part and make it more difficult to manage, you can still manage this type of high cholesterol as you would any other type, with diet and lifestyle changes, and as a last resort, with medications.

Do not confuse the fact that 95% of your cholesterol is made by your own body with the incidence of high cholesterol as a genetic tendency. As mentioned above, the numbers indicate that in the US and most other countries, the incidence is about 1 person in 500, or .02%. If you suspect you are one of them, gather as much family medical history as possible, especially in your direct line, and consult your doctor about blood testing. Also, do not disregard the fact that families tend to have similar diet and lifestyle, both of which are factors in developing or not developing high cholesterol levels. Even if your family history reveals a pattern of hypercholesterolemia and even if you have an inherited genetic mutation, you can break the stereotypical family patterns of dining on foods high in saturated fat, lack of exercise, weight issues and substance (particularly alcohol and tobacco) abuse that characterize the lifestyle most likely to result in high cholesterol.

However, as we have hinted already, high cholesterol in and of itself is not the problem, but rather, merely a symptom of the problem.

# Honing in on the real villain - oxidized cholesterol

You may be familiar with oxidation in the form of fruit that turns brown shortly after being cut. The process is a chemical one, and it occurs naturally in your body as it assimilates oxygen. You may have heard and wondered about the term 'free radical', so let's talk about this chemical reaction a bit. Without getting too scientific, chemical reactions happen when one atom or molecule combines with another, sometimes knocking off bits or pieces of each of the combined units.  The chemical reactions happening continuously within your body are collectively called metabolism, which you may have thought was the process of burning calories. In fact, it means the process of combining oxygen with your cells to generate or regenerate them, constantly renewing dead cells to keep your marvelously complex machine running. That could also be considered as burning, and the calories you count are an expression of the fuel required to keep those cells in constant regeneration. In the normal course of things, your body is very efficient at metabolizing oxygen; however, about 1%-2% of the time, this process knocks off a bit of another molecule and leaves what you can picture as a sharp edge, a free radical, hanging off it.

Free radicals are unstable molecules that need another electron to become stable. You could picture a jigsaw puzzle piece run amok, bumping into other pieces to try to fill that hole with an electron, and in the process knocking off bits of the other pieces in a chain reaction that could cause a lot of damage to the puzzle as a whole; in other words, oxidation. Fortunately, there are counter-terrorism substances called antioxidants. The word literally means 'against oxidation.' Mother Nature has provided us with the perfect defense within our food, because several vitamins and micro-nutrients willingly give up their electrons to stabilize the free radicals. If we get enough of these antioxidants, our bodies can minimize the damage.

Going back to the damage that is caused by free radicals, though, we have taken a rather simplistic look at it. If it were that simple, the answer would be simple as well. To return to our analogy, when a free radical knocks a bit off of another molecule. it may not be simply a matter of the damaged molecule needing to find another electron. The bit that got knocked off might be part of the DNA, or the instruction code for what function that cell is supposed to perform within your body. When the cell gets replicated or regenerated with damaged DNA, it will be making a faulty copy of itself. Have you ever seen a third- or fourth-generation fax document? It gets fuzzier and fuzzier as the copies multiply, eventually becoming unreadable. In the same way, cells with damaged DNA get further and further from their optimal state. Some even begin to rapidly multiply, causing cancer among other things.

If you have excess cholesterol circulating in your bloodstream, some of it might be laid down along the walls of your arteries as your blood passes through them. If the oxidative process described above happens within these deposits, it can cause blockages that prevents blood from passing through the arteries as it should. If that happens in an artery that leads to your heart, the resulting deprivation of oxygen to your heart will cause a heart attack. If it happens within arteries leading to your brain, it causes stroke. You can see how medical researchers have formed the conclusion that it is the excess cholesterol that is the problem. However, it is the oxidation of that cholesterol that causes the ultimate problem.

You may be asking, "If the problem is free radicals and we can fight those with antioxidants, why is there a problem?" The answer to that lies in the fact that there are many environmental factors that create free radicals, and those factors are increasing all the time. From toxins in the air and on our food, to those we voluntarily allow inside our bodies, like cigarette smoke and alcohol, the oxidative burden of modern man is much higher than it was a few generations ago. Certainly, some have always been around. But our lifestyle as modern people, with chemicals surrounding us in our air-tight homes, less exercise and more highly processed foods, auto exhaust and industrial pollution, causes us to encounter more than our grandparents and great-grandparents did. At the same time, we now rely less on fresh foods with antioxidant properties and more on highly processed, often deep-fried, fast food. Even those of us who try to incorporate fresh fruit and vegetables in our diets are getting less than what we think we are, as foods that have been imported from distant locations have less nutritional value due to losses in transit.

"So," you may say, "how does that translate to free radicals in my body, and more importantly, oxidation damaging my cholesterol?"

## How Does Cholesterol Get Oxidized?

To understand the answer to this question, we need to understand a little bit about the body's natural defenses. You may already know that when you become ill or injured, the white cells of your blood rush to the area of illness to attack the invading germ or virus. Red cells follow quickly to bring needed oxygen to the area so that the white cells and other blood cells that have their own specific purposes can be replenished. Some of those other cells are called macrophages, and their purpose is to consume the dead germ cells. The red cells rushing in is what causes the redness around a cut or scrape, the fever you experience when fighting an infection, and other evidence that your body's natural defenses are on the job. This is called inflammation, another way to describe the 'burning', i.e., oxidation, that is taking place as each cell calls on replacement reserves of oxygen to do its job. When it is defending you from external attack, inflammation is a good thing. However, it can also be dangerous, as we will see.

Previously, we discussed cholesterol collecting in the arteries when there is too much of it in the bloodstream. Actually, it is not that simple. You might have pictured it just falling out of suspension in the bloodstream like the snowflakes in a snow globe that fall to the bottom when you stop shaking it, piling up in the artery and forming a sort of dam that blocks the blood flow. That is not the way it happens, though. In fact, it is attracted to and incorporated into the walls of the artery. The lining of the blood vessels have a characteristically smooth structure, but when damaged by inflammation they can become sticky. This happens because of a chemical reaction induced by inflammation, but it typically does not block the artery by itself. What blocks the artery is a blood clot that is formed when the plaque ruptures within the artery walls due to inflammation.
Here is a more detailed description of how that happens: In the presence of oxidative stress or high blood sugar, LDL (the substance that carries cholesterol through the bloodstream and into the cells) is chemically changed, and those changes are perceived by your immune system to be dangerous. As a result, it rushes defender cells to the area, which in turn "roughs up" the smooth cell walls with what has been called a Velcro effect. Imagine all the little hooks that hold the loops of the opposite side of Velcro. Those little hooks are similar to the rough areas inside the blood vessel walls that make them 'sticky'. The macrophages, perceiving the altered LDL to be an infectious agent, gobble it up and become fat themselves, eventually dying and leaving what is called the lipid core, a fatty residue often called foam cells, which are also living cells. This process is what deposits the cholesterol within the artery walls, and would not happen without the inflammation that chemically changes the LDL.

Fascinating as this is, it is all happening where we cannot see it! Only during surgery or autopsy can this story be read. Dr. Lunden, whose previously-quoted book gives a very extensive description of the process that I have summarized here, describes a vicious cycle, during which the body's defensive cells release toxins of their own that create further damage and attract more defensive cells to contain it. Eventually this process so degenerates the artery wall that the plaque ruptures, and the body responds by containing what it perceives to be a foreign substance by forming a blood clot, essentially a scab, over it. When that clot blocks the blood flow, whatever is beyond that point that depends on the oxygen the blood is carrying begins to die. Whether your body dies suddenly from this event or not depends largely on the location of the blockage.

The good news is that if you can interrupt the inflammation before it gets to this dire conclusion, your body will actually form a protective fibrous cap over the plaque, stabilizing it and preventing rupture in the absence of new inflammation. To interrupt the inflammation, you must understand the role of all the factors that generate it and take control of them. Medicine won't do it; however, if you are already taking medicine for high cholesterol, you must not under any circumstances stop taking it without your doctor's knowledge and cooperation. The advice to come in the remainder of this book will help you prevent or eliminate inflammation, which will make you healthier in general. You will probably want to discuss lowering or eliminating your medication with your doctor afterward.

# Inflammation and Cholesterol

At this point, you may be wondering what causes all this inflammation in the first place. We'll start with the obvious, and go from there. Earlier we discussed some of the risk factors for heart disease that had been identified by the Framingham Study, other than high cholesterol. Would it surprise you by now to know that many of them contribute to inflammation in your body? Let's look at them one by one.

## Smoking

We all know what kind of damage smoking does to our lungs, and yet many cling to whatever benefit they perceive they get from it, assuming the health bill from it will not come due for many years. What if they knew that with every inhalation, chemicals from smoke were not only introducing carcinogens into the lungs that may or may not eventually cause cancer, but were also infusing the blood stream with toxins that cause inflammation? If you are a smoker, think about when you first started smoking, how irritating the smoke was to your throat. Every drag from a cigarette continues to cause the same kind of irritation to the walls of the blood vessels when the chemicals from smoke are carried there by the bloodstream. We just discussed what happens when the interior of the blood cells become irritated — smoking causes the oxidative stress that starts the process. The way to reduce inflammation from smoking is simple: stop smoking, and stay well away from second-hand smoke, which is possibly even more detrimental.

## High Blood Pressure

Also known as hypertension, this health condition is a symptom of several other conditions, but in and of itself it damages the blood vessels. Hypertension is associated with high levels of angiotensin, a potent vasoconstrictor. Angiotensin is a peptide hormone whose role in the body is to constrict blood vessels under certain conditions when that is desirable, such as when your body needs to form a blood clot over a wound. Various forms also play other roles within other body systems, such as acting in such a way as to increase the desire for salt or increasing thirst. While we identify an excess of it with constricting artery walls and causing high blood pressure, it is important to remember that it, like cholesterol, is a natural part of the body's complex checks and balances. When it is busy causing problems, however, it does so by initiating the Velcro effect changes mentioned above.

It is interesting to note that an effect of obesity is that fat cells produce a pre-cursor to angiotensin. The excess production of angiotensin causes a feedback loop, wherein hypertension becomes both a cause and a result of hypertension. As it progresses, the blood vessel deteriorates and stiffens, further constricting it so that it cannot accommodate increased blood flow when necessary, leading to more high blood pressure and so on until tragedy strikes.

The way to reduce inflammation from high blood pressure is obviously to lower it; however that subject is complex in its own right. Suffice it to say that reducing external stressors, losing weight and exercising are all parts of the equation.

## Elevated Blood Sugar

It used to be thought that eating sugar and simple carbohydrates would cause diabetes. Then the medical profession said no, that was not the cause, but it would exacerbate the effects of a shortage of insulin or of insulin resistance, which is a learned response of the cells in the presence of elevated blood sugar wherein the cells do not properly utilize the insulin that is present. Coming full circle, we now know that consuming excessive amounts of refined sugar and simple carbohydrates acts in two ways to contribute to developing Type II diabetes. The first is that sugar and simple carbs are high in calories, but low in factors that cause satiety. So we eat far too many of them to try to feel less hungry. The more we eat, the more calories we have to burn off to avoid getting fatter.

This then leads to another of those vicious cycles: we eat more sugar, we still feel hungry and we don't feel enough energy to work off the calories, so we get fat. Meanwhile, our pancreas is working overtime to produce enough insulin, which is the hormone tasked with shoving fuel in the form of blood sugar into the cells where it is either stored or used. When you consume sugars and simple carbs (which are broken down into sugars in your blood stream), it is easy for the insulin to sweep it out of the bloodstream at first, especially in the absence of anything like fiber, fat and protein to slow it down. When your pancreas is working overtime to produce large amounts of insulin, the first result is hypoglycemia, or low blood sugar, the result of that excess insulin shoving ALL of your fuel into storage and leaving none for your body to work with for current needs.

Like shoving too much paperwork in your desk drawer, eventually that stops working because there is no more room. At that point you have what is called insulin resistance. The cells will no longer open to receive the blood sugar, and that is the beginning of Type II diabetes. As long as your body detects excess blood sugar it will try to produce the insulin needed to put it away, so to speak. Eventually, the pancreas is worn out and you have full-blown, insulin-dependent, Type II diabetes. But how does this relate to heart disease? High blood sugar irritates the lining of the arteries, causing them to be inflamed. Once again we have conditions for cholesterol to collect in them and potentially rupture.

Rather than giving a simple answer to reducing inflammation from elevated blood sugar, which is another complex subject, let us leave it at 'consume less sugar and simple carbohydrates.' While that may not be the whole answer, it is at least a start. In later sections we will discuss the essential components of an anti-inflammatory eating plan and present a few recipes that will show you how a few simple changes will both lower your dependence on sugar and simple carbs and provide you with a tastier alternative.

## Consuming the wrong fats

You may have heard the phrase 'good fat' versus the phrase 'bad fat'. You may even know that highly saturated fats or trans-fats are the bad kind, while vegetable oils, fish oil and fats from certain fruits (like avocado) are the good kind. In reality, it is not that simple. While it is certainly the case that trans-fats are bad and to be avoided at all costs, not all saturated fats are bad and not all vegetable oils are created equal.

Most trans-fats are artificial compounds created by hydrogenating (literally, incorporating hydrogen into) vegetable oils. This creates shortening, margarine and other substances that are found nowhere in nature. The 'trans' part of the descriptive word comes from the fact that the molecule thus created is backwards from the molecules of fats that are naturally solid at room temperature. Your body literally does not know what to do with these molecules, which causes havoc when you consume them. Among other things, they interfere with the absorption of Omega-3 fatty acids (the really good kind of fat) and have been shown to increase C-reactive protein, the marker for chronic low-grade inflammation.

Animal fats like the marbling you find in good-quality beef, the layer underneath chicken and turkey skin, butter and rendered pig fat (lard) are all saturated fats. All of this type of fat is solid at room temperature, and most of it is good for only one thing: it tastes good. Our bodies evolved, depending on the locations where our ancestors roamed, consuming some saturated fat. The operative word here is 'some.' It was difficult for hunter-gatherers to bring home animals to eat, unlike now when we can go and 'hunt' our meat at the supermarket. Even when they did have a good kill, as likely or not the animal was quite lean, as it was not raised in a feed lot where it was stuffed with grain and hormones to make it bigger and fatter. Today we consume far too much of it because it is readily available...and because it tastes good.

Further complicating the picture are the Omega-6 versus Omega-3 essential fatty acids and Mono-unsaturated versus Poly-unsaturated fats. Both monounsaturated and polyunsaturated fats are considered 'good' fats. The difference is in the molecular structure, but what you really need to know is what foods contain each, which we will get to in later sections. Likewise, both Omega-6 and Omega-3 fats are good for you, when consumed in the right proportions. Again, you need to know which foods contain which in order to consume them in the right proportions, and again we will get to that in later chapters. For now, let's talk about that 'right proportions' phrase.

Dr. Andrew Weil, a noted American physician whose focus is on healthy eating, has stated in his writing that in our past, even up to recent times before we started relying so heavily on prepared and highly processed foods, human beings naturally consumed roughly equal proportions of each of these types of fat. Now, however, the Omega-6 type is far more prevalent in our diets. Furthermore, it is a fact that when we are digesting these nutrients Omega-6 fatty acids tend to metabolize into more pro-inflammatory compounds, while Omega-3 fatty acids tend to metabolize into more anti-inflammatory compounds. This means that if they are consumed in the right proportions they would balance each other out, but our modern diets have us eating in such a way that we create far more inflammatory compounds than the anti-inflammatory ones can balance.

Let's go back for a moment to the names of these fats that is 'essential fatty acids'. Why is that word essential in the name? It is because they are necessary to life and health, but we cannot make them for ourselves, as we can other types of fats, within our bodies. We must consume them. So equally important in the equation are two rules: consuming less Omega-6 and more Omega-3 will double your anti-inflammatory efforts. See the anti-inflammatory eating plan later in this book for foods to look for in both categories.

## Stress

Unless you have had your head in the sand for the last decade, you already know that external stressors contribute to the manufacture in your body of the hormone cortisol. Less widely known is the role of cytokines, a multifunctional protein that plays a role in cell communication and activation. Both of these substances are beneficial to the body in their proper roles, but an excess or constantly-circulating level is counterproductive. "What could possibly be a good role for cortisol," you may ask. Well, if you were one of your hunter ancestors, you would probably be able to answer that for yourself. Cortisol is involved in the release of adrenaline, the 'fight or flight' hormone. Nevertheless, we did not evolve to handle the chronic, constant stress we are subjected to in our modern world. This chronic stress has been shown to increase the levels of cytokines in the bloodstream, and the cytokines also initiate the previously discussed Velcro effect on the arteries.

Physical stress such as chronic pain can have the same effect. Some of our stress cannot be avoided, but much of it is self-inflicted. Lowering your stress levels will assist with eliminating chronic inflammation.

## Obesity

We have already discussed obesity as it relates to Type II diabetes. However, in addition to that factor, obesity brings a couple of other inflammatory circumstances into play. The first is the toxins that are easily stored in our fat cells, some of them the wrong kinds of fat that we discussed earlier. Excess fat also leads to excess LDL in our bloodstreams—the type of cholesterol that is stored within the artery walls. Are you beginning to see the complex interactions of all our body processes that create the vicious cycle? In addition to these problems, obesity leads to chronic pain, one of the stressors that we can absolutely control by losing that excess weight and taking the burden off our joints, tendons and ligaments.

## Vitamin Deficiency

Consuming the wrong kinds of fat, the wrong proportions of the right kinds of fat and too much refined carbohydrates are not the only food-related damage we are doing to ourselves. Several vitamins are known to be anti-inflammatory and deficiencies in those vitamins prevent our bodies from protecting themselves. Among them are vitamins A, C and E. Vitamin D, which you may know as the sunshine vitamin, was once thought to be important only to bone health and absorption of calcium. It is now known to be a powerful anti-microbial, anti-cancer and anti-inflammatory as well.

We are deficient in these vitamins for several reasons, but the main one is that we are starving ourselves of nutrients while making ourselves obese with too much of the wrong kinds of food. Do you remember when your mother said to you, "Don't eat those cookies right now, you'll spoil your dinner?" Did you think that you could ignore that advice once you grew up and were responsible for your own diet? It was sound advice! Yet, Eric Schlosser wrote in Fast Food Nation, "Over the last three decades, fast food has infiltrated every nook and cranny of American society. An industry that began with a handful of modest hot dog and hamburger stands in southern California has spread to every corner of the nation, selling a broad range of foods wherever paying customers may be found. Fast food is now served at restaurants and drive-throughs, at stadiums, airports, zoos, high schools, elementary schools, and universities, on cruise ships, trains, and airplanes, at K-Marts, Wal-Marts, gas stations, and even at hospital cafeterias. In 1970, Americans spent about $6 billion on fast food; in 2000, they spent more than $110 billion. Americans now spend more money on fast food than on higher education, personal computers, computer software, or new cars. They spend more on fast food than on movies, books, magazines, newspapers, videos, and recorded music combined."

Although fast food chains have recently made an effort to be perceived as offering more healthy food choices, the fact is that when presented with a choice between a tasty, 1000-calorie bacon cheeseburger and a mediocre salad, most Americans will choose the cheeseburger. Those that choose the salad may be appalled to discover that if they put that packet of salad dressing on it, it could well represent the same number of calories, while offering the dubious nutrients of mostly iceberg lettuce and a few shreds of carrots, topped with fried chicken, cheese and other foods just as high in saturated fats as the cheeseburger. Who wants a healthy meal after that calorie-bomb?

Furthermore, modern convenience foods like canned goods, frozen vegetable offerings topped with heavy sauces and deli salads full of mayonnaise, sour cream or the like have all replaced the fresh, simple produce that was found on your ancestors' tables or around their campfires. Why do we take a perfectly healthy sweet potato, practically no fat, full of fiber and potassium and 184 calories per cup when baked, and turn it into something that would be more at home on a dessert menu—sweet potato casserole, 460 calories or more, full of fat, with half the fiber and more than twice the sugars as served at one popular restaurant chain? Because we have forgotten how to taste real food and crave instead the salt, sugar and fat that we associate with 'good flavor.' All of this stuff that's bad for us is preventing us from being hungry for the nutrients that are good for us, including vitamins. However, vitamin supplementation is not the answer! Excess amounts of the vitamins we began this discussion with can be toxic. We need to return to our foods the natural amounts of vitamins and minerals they had in bygone times, and consume our nutrients the way we evolved to consume them.

## Anti-inflammatory medications

One would think that if our heart disease epidemic is a matter of chronic inflammation as much as high cholesterol, that applying anti-inflammatory medications to the problem would make it go away. And yet, what is actually happening is a rebound effect, where our bodies stop making the anti-inflammatory proteins and hormones themselves, and become reliant on the medications instead. Nor are these medications without other risks, as you can clearly see if you read a list of their side-effects. Any time you upset the delicate balance of chemicals within your body, you are going to see adverse effects. You may be familiar with some of them if you were ever on the COX-2inhibitor class of anti-inflammatory medication Vioxx. COX 2 is a natural enzyme that has an important function in the body. Inhibiting its manufacture will reduce inflammation; however, it will also (through a complex chain of chemical process) constrict the blood vessels, leading to blood clots and stroke. For this reason, Vioxx has been taken off the market, along with another medication of its class. At this time, the only brand-name COX-2 inhibitor still on the market in the US is Celebrex.

Of all the anti-inflammatory medications on the market, only the oldest and least understood in terms of how it works— aspirin— makes blood platelets less sticky and does not lead to clotting. In fact, aspirin leads to the opposite problem, but that is for another discussion.

All of these factors are to some extent, some more, some less, in our control. We have the power to change our bad habits, our weight, and our diets. In many ways these are all connected to each other, as with our bad eating habits leading to obesity and obesity being related to Type II diabetes and so forth. Other than smoking and some of the external stressors in our lives, in fact, all of these concerns can be directly affected, and improved, by improving the way we eat. In the next section, we will take up the discussion of specific changes you can make to eliminate inflammation through your diet.

# The Anti-Inflammation Diet

Do not confuse the eating plan we are about to introduce with the standard diet to lower cholesterol. Many of the recommendations may be the same; however the intent is to attack the real problem rather than the perceived problem. We have already discussed the anti-inflammatory properties of certain fats, and the importance of balancing those fats in the proper proportions. We have talked about the anti-inflammatory vitamins A, C, D and E. Now let's talk about how to incorporate these important substances into our lives on a daily basis through the foods we eat.

## Trans-fats

If you are consuming the typical American diet that is high in fat, particularly the 'bad' saturated and trans-fats associated with fast food, red meat, whole dairy and prepared baked goods, the first place to begin improving your diet is here. WebMD mentions that the worst of the worst are artificial trans-fats, i.e., partially-hydrogenated vegetable oils, otherwise known as shortening. This is the type of fat that has been under attack in the fast-food industry, where it was once used exclusively for fries, fried chicken and the like. However, you may not know that it is also to be found in biscuit mix, pie shells, crackers, bakery goods and some margarines. Some trans fats are also naturally-occurring, in animal fat for example, but they don't seem to be as harmful as the artificial type that are made by adding hydrogen to vegetable oils. The harmful effects of partially-hydrogenated oils include raising LDL, lowering HDL and contributing to inflammation, a triple-whammy that you can avoid by simply paying attention to food labels. Does this mean you must never again enjoy any of the foods mentioned above? Not necessarily. Many fast-food restaurants have responded to criticism by substituting other oils for their frying, and if you bake at home you can do the same.

It could be helpful for you to take note of the food labels on foods you normally enjoy, and jot down how many servings times how much trans-fats in grams you are consuming. Be aware that if a serving of a food contains less than .5 grams of trans-fat, manufacturers are legally able to label it as 0; however, that adds up if you have several servings a day, or if you are unaware of what a serving actually is. Always read labels, and find the nutritional information for your favorite fast foods online or on in-store posters. Your target consumption of trans-fats should be less than 1% of your daily caloric intake.

## Other Saturated Fats

Saturated fats other than artificial trans-fats include animal fat (particularly that found in red meat or lard), dairy (including cream, butter, cheese and all milk other than skim), poultry and poultry skin, coconut products, palm oil and palm kernel oil and associated products. These are the next target on your improvement list. The 2010 Dietary Guidelines promulgated by the USDA recommend limiting saturated fats to 10% or less of your total calories, while the American Heart Association recommends keeping them to just 7% of total calories.

It is not at all difficult to avoid some of these products simply by lowering your dependence on red meat in favor of poultry, and making sure you do not consume the skin of the latter. Adding some vegetarian favorites and at least three servings of cold-water fish a week will further improve the saturated fat picture.

Wean yourself from whole milk by gradually mixing in more and more 2% until you are drinking just 2%, and then repeat with 1% and on to skim. There are several products on the market that lower the saturated fat content of butter by mixing in buttermilk or canola oil, although these are less satisfactory for baking or cooking. However, you can substitute olive oil in most of your cooking, and there are many recipes for baked goods that substitute fat-free applesauce for some or all of the oil called for in traditional recipes. See the recipe section for a few favorites. Finally, opt for the lower-fat or fat-free versions of sour cream, cottage cheese and cream cheese. These are easily found, work fine in recipes and taste fine as well. If you do not find them to your liking at first, use the gradual method suggested for milk to re-set your taste buds' expectations.

Consume other cheeses sparingly, as there are few really satisfactory substitutes on the market. Those that vegans and some vegetarians have found satisfactory are often made with soy. If you can tolerate soy products and find these to your taste, they are preferable for the purpose of lowering intake of saturated fats.

## Mono-unsaturated fats

These are the so-called 'good' fats, found in olives; avocados; hazelnuts; almonds; Brazil nuts; cashews; sesame seeds; pumpkin seeds; and olive, canola, and peanut oils. MUFAs became the darling of the healthy weight-loss gurus with the discovery that heart disease is lower in Mediterranean countries, it is thought because of their high reliance on olive oil in the diet. With regard to our anti-inflammatory diet, however, we must note that Americans now consume a higher proportion of these fats than is optimal. It is not usually necessary to add foods high in these fats, as we get sufficient MUFAs if we are consuming healthy choices. Nevertheless, for cooking with oil, olive, canola and peanut oils remain the gold standard, as the polyunsaturated oils are unable to withstand high heat.

Certainly snacks of the above-mentioned nuts and seeds are preferable to the potato chips and pre-packaged snacks that we consume without thought; however we must also be mindful of the high caloric content in them. Because obesity is essentially an inflammatory condition, it does no good to eliminate bad fats and substitute good ones if we are going to consume 35% or more of our calories from fat (a recent estimate of current American fat consumption).

## Poly-unsaturated fats

These are the fats that we need to increase in our diets, again being mindful of the calories involved. They are also possibly some of the most difficult to integrate into the typical American diet. The food highest in the Omega-3 family of poly-unsaturated fatty acids is flax oil, an oil that cannot be used in cooking and must be refrigerated to remain fresh. Flax oil has a nutty taste and a slightly bitter aftertaste that becomes more pronounced as the freshness diminishes.

The next highest Omega-3 containing food is flax seeds, followed closely by certain types of fish oil (salmon being at the top of the list) and the fish themselves. Walnuts, walnut oil and oddly, Chinese broccoli along with several herbs and spices make the top 50. Obviously the herbs and spices are going to be the least useful as they are consumed in such small quantities, although basil - the primary ingredient in pesto - is one of them.

It is incumbent upon us, as we take responsibility for our own health, to try new foods and find new ways of incorporating these foods into our diets. Nutritionists recommend that we get our Omega-3s from the foods we eat rather than supplements; however, supplementation is better than not getting them at all, as long as we pay attention to recommended doses. From www.mayoclinic.com :

*There is supportive evidence from multiple studies that suggests the intake of recommended amounts of DHA and EPA in the form of dietary fish or fish oil supplements lowers triglycerides; reduces the risk of death, heart attack, dangerous abnormal heart rhythms, and strokes in people with known cardiovascular disease; slows the buildup of atherosclerotic plaques ("hardening of the arteries"), and lowers blood pressure slightly. However, high doses may have harmful effects, such as an increased risk of bleeding.*

# Foods high in Vitamin A

Before we get to the foods highest in vitamin A, we must caution you that it is not only possible but easy to overdose on this vitamin, turning it from a beneficial ingredient in your diet to a detrimental one, potentially leading to jaundice, nausea, loss of appetite, irritability, vomiting, and hair loss. The current RDA for Vitamin A is 5000 international units (IU).

The top ten foods that are high in vitamin A starts with one that may not be first on your favorite foods list: liver. All animal liver is high in vitamin A, as is cod liver oil. A single tablespoon of pâté will provide 429 IU (9% RDA) of vitamin A, and a teaspoon of cod liver oil will provide 500IU (10% RDA). However, liver is also a source of high dietary cholesterol. If you have familial hypercholesterolemia or if your doctor insists you maintain a low-cholesterol diet, it would be best to obtain your vitamin A from other foods. Next come spicy-hot red peppers and the spices made from them: paprika, cayenne and chili powder. In fact, a red or orange color is associated with the vegetables and fruits highest in vitamin A: red and orange bell pepper, sweet potatoes, carrots, butternut squash, dried apricots and cantaloupe. Dark green and red leafy lettuce is also among the top ten, as are most herbs. This variety gives us a great start in adding healthful, low-fat, highly nutritious anti-inflammatory foods to our diet. In the recipe section, you will find recipes for many of these vegetables that will please your taste buds as well as fight inflammation.

# Foods high in Vitamin C

Vitamin C is important to several functions in the body, including the development and maintenance of blood vessels, protective (scar) tissue, and cartilage as well as some essential amino acids and hormones. As a powerful anti-inflammatory substance, vitamin C helps lessen oxidative stress to the body and is thought to lower cancer risk. And of course, everyone 'knows' that vitamin C shortens the course of colds, if not preventing them altogether — if you believe anecdotal evidence.

You may think of orange juice as your top source of vitamin C, but in fact oranges are only #9 on the list of the top ten sources. Heading that list are red and green chili peppers, which provide several times the 60 mg current RDA in just half a cup of chopped pepper. Guava is next on the list, followed by bell peppers of all colors and several dark green leafy vegetables: parsley, thyme, kale, mustard greens, garden cress and broccoli. Next come several fruits: in order of highest to lowest, kiwi, papaya, oranges and strawberries. Of all the anti-oxidant vitamins, C is the only one that is water-soluble and must therefore be replenished daily. The rest are fat-soluble, so they are stored in your body if excess amounts are provided either through your diet or supplementation.

# Foods high in Vitamin D

Once thought to be important only in assisting calcium in bone maintenance, we now know that vitamin D is a potent anti-carcinogenic, anti-microbial and yes, anti-inflammatory substance. Deficiency in vitamin D can lead to rickets, a disease of the bones in which they fail to properly develop. It can also lead to a weakened immune system, osteomalacia, a condition of weakened muscles and bones, and increased cancer risk. On the other hand, excess vitamin D can cause the body to absorb too much calcium, which has been related to both heart attacks and kidney stones. The current U.S. DV for vitamin D is 600 IU (international units) and the toxicity threshold for vitamin D is thought to be 10,000 to 40,000 IU/day. For this reason alone, it is preferable to get our vitamin D from the food we eat rather than from supplementation.

You may recall that vitamin D is called the sunshine vitamin, because your body makes it when you expose your skin to the sun. About 15 minutes a day of natural sunlight on skin that does not have sunscreen applied is sufficient for most people to make all they need. However, with the concern about skin cancer causing most Americans to liberally apply sunscreen and the prevalence of indoor entertainments keeping our outdoor time to a minimum, it is also a good idea to eat some foods high in vitamin D to make sure you get enough. Vitamin D is commonly added to milk and orange juice, but if you don't consume these, get yours from the following ten foods.

First on the list is our old friend cod liver oil, followed by several types of fatty fish including salmon and mackerel as well as oil-packed tuna and sardines. Raw fish is higher in vitamin D than cooked, and canned fish packed in oil is higher in vitamin D than that packed in water. Do be careful when consuming raw fish, as environmental toxins are increasingly present. Certain fortified cereals come next, but again you must exercise caution as you could be trading that healthful vitamin D for too much sugar and partially-hydrogenated vegetable oils, both commonly found in processed cereals—be sure to read the label. Next come oysters, which are high in cholesterol and not recommended for people whose cholesterol levels mandate a low-cholesterol diet. Following that is caviar, both black and red. If those foods are not your favorite, consider fortified soy products, including tofu and soy milk, again if you are able to tolerate soy products. Soy is contra-indicated if you have impaired thyroid function, however. Next come salami, ham and sausage. These, too, have their problems, being high in both fat and sodium. The final three are eggs, certain mushrooms and dairy products, which often are fortified with vitamin D so as to make the most of the calcium found in them, but also have natural vitamin D,.

## Foods high in Vitamin E

Vitamin E is actually a group of eight vitamins that help prevent heart disease, macular degeneration and cancer through anti-oxidant action. Like A and D, E is fat-soluble, so it is better to get it from food than supplementation that can lead to getting too much. Excess vitamin E can cause hemorrhaging. The following foods are considered to have safe amounts of vitamin E when consumed in moderation.

Sunflower seeds get top billing, with paprika and red chili powder in second. However, it would require about 7 tablespoons of either spice to get the full RDA of vitamin E. Almonds, either in raw form as a snack or in almond butter or almond milk, provide the next highest amount of vitamin E per serving, and pine nuts are next. Also high in vitamin E are peanuts, dried herbs (basil and oregano), dried apricots, pickled green olives, cooked spinach, and cooked taro root. If you are unfamiliar with taro, it is a tuber that is inedible raw, but a good substitute for potatoes when baked or boiled, or it can be made into bread. It is a staple in some countries, most notably Polynesian countries and Asia. You can find it in Asian markets if not in your local grocery.

You may have noticed that several foods are high in more than one of the anti-oxidant vitamins, or that some seem to suggest dishes where more than one of them can be combined to get all four vitamins. Be sure to check the recipe section for some suggestions to make sure you get adequate amounts daily.

## Putting it all together

Like any 'diet', in the sense of a structured food plan that radically changes your habits, you may consider an anti-inflammatory diet to be a lot of work, and possibly somewhat pricey, at first. However, you must weigh the benefits also to determine whether you will make an effort to change or not. If you have ever been on a weight-reduction diet, you know that it is not possible to deprive yourself of your favorite foods 'cold turkey' and long-term unless you have a life-threatening condition that requires such a drastic change. Even then, some people find their will-power to be insufficient to the task. If you have not already been diagnosed with dangerous levels of cholesterol, atherosclerosis or serious heart disease, you may find it easier and more long-lasting to gradually alter your eating habits to conform to an anti-inflammatory diet. However, your own situation will determine whether you will adopt an anti-inflammatory diet whole-heartedly or more gradually change your eating habits to allow you to adjust your preferences to the healthier choices. Bear in mind that heart disease and stroke are often silent killers, striking the fatal blow without previous warning. If you have read the causes of inflammation with alarm, realizing your lifestyle has included all of them, you might consider that you already have or may have a life-threatening condition that has not yet made itself known.

If you are attempting to reduce your inflammation and lower your LDL quickly, the 'jump in with both feet' method will have the best chance of doing that, but may also require you to adjust to some feelings of deprivation. If you are able to apply discipline and time to the outcome, the gradual method may be best for you. No matter which method you choose, you will find the table of foods to avoid and foods to add or substitute at the end of this book a vital resource to take with you while grocery shopping. You will also need to determine whether you should lose weight while consuming anti-inflammatory foods or not.

There are several published diets that either claim to be anti-inflammatory or are similar to those that make the claim. One is Dr. Andrew Weil's Anti-Inflammatory pyramid and diet, which we will explore in more detail below. According to US News & World Report, it is similar to others, including the Flexitarian Diet, the Mediterranean Diet and several more. The key similarity seems to be a heavy emphasis on vegetables and fruits, nuts and seeds, whole grains and moderate amounts (if any) of animal protein. As mentioned above, any of these may have rules that are rigid or difficult to follow and most have either too little of certain nutrients or too much sodium. However, they are a good start in your journey, as long as you pay attention to the deficiencies of the published diet and modify it to meet your individual requirements.

# Dr. Weil's Anti-Inflammatory Pyramid

Dr. Andrew Weil is a noted American medical doctor who pioneered the field of integrative medicine, which he describes as blending Western medicine with alternative therapies such as exercise, spiritual practice and most of all, nutrition. Weil recommends that patients take the medication that their doctors give them, and then add the alternative therapies. While he has been roundly criticized by some in the medical profession, his theories and philosophies appeal widely to his audience. Even sceptics have to admit that some, perhaps many, of his theories have been subsequently proven or supported by independent medical research, such as the notion that general, chronic inflammation in the body is responsible for or implicated in a variety of serious illnesses. Dr. Weil has long been a proponent of a diet heavily weighted with fruits and vegetables, preferably organic, fish and Omega-3 fatty acids to combat the condition of chronic inflammation. His reduction of what could otherwise be a confusing array of nutritional advice to the familiar pyramid analogy is instructive as our guide to a diet to eliminate chronic inflammation.

Beginning at the bottom with the foods you should choose the most of, we find fruits and vegetables. Dr. Weil suggests 4-5 a day minimum of the latter and 3-4 a day minimum of the former, both fresh and frozen, using a variety of colors and choosing organic if possible. Conversely, the Mediterranean diet (which is touted as a weight-loss diet rather than one for reducing inflammation per se) urges users to avoid fruits because they have a high sugar content and are therefore higher in calories than are vegetables. If you wish to lose weight on your anti-inflammatory diet, you might do well to substitute an equal number of vegetables for fruit—over and above the recommended number of vegetables in the pyramid. While choosing your fruits and vegetables, remember those that are highest in the anti-inflammatory vitamins. A serving of vegetables is typically set at ½ cup, but may be more for vegetables that are particularly high in water content, in which case a whole vegetable might be a serving. An example of the latter might be cucumber. A serving of fruit is usually a whole or half fruit, except in the case of melons or other very large fruits, in which case the serving might be ½-1 cup. Although we would not typically eat less than a whole banana, count a medium to large banana as two servings.

The next layer of the pyramid consists of the foods that will provide both protein and the fiber that will help you feel full and satisfied as well as keeping your waste disposal functions running smoothly. Remember that inflammation can occur from a sluggish elimination system, also. Fiber is vital to a healthy diet, so we will take this opportunity to reiterate that the current popularity of low- or no-carb diets is targeting the wrong aspect of this class of macronutrients. What is unhealthful is highly processed carbohydrates with the fiber removed; for example, white flour, white rice, refined and heavily sugared prepared cereal. Instead, choose 3-5 servings a day of whole and cracked grains, bearing in mind that a serving is usually ½ to ¾ of a cup, not an entire bowlful. Also found in this layer are beans and legumes, of which you should consume 1 or 2 servings a day. Again, a serving is ½ to ¾ cup. Two or three times a week, you may enjoy a serving of pasta, but be sure to choose those that are made with whole grains rather than refined flours. You will find the whole grains to be more flavorful, and any distaste you may have for the texture after spending your entire previous life consuming the refined varieties will soon be overcome through familiarity.

You may be pleasantly surprised to find the healthy fats at the next level of the pyramid. Depending on whether you are looking at Dr. Weil's recommendations, those of the USDA or of the American Heart Association, anywhere from 15-35% of your daily caloric needs should come from fats. Fats are essential to the breakdown and assimilation of three of the four anti-inflammatory vitamins as well as other vital bodily functions; and besides that, they taste good. Remember again to choose those with the highest anti-inflammatory properties as listed above, and avoid those that contribute to inflammation. Dr. Weil's pyramid recommends 5-7 servings per day, using as examples the following list: extra-virgin olive oil, impeller-expressed canola oil, nuts (especially walnuts), and seeds including hemp seeds (high in protein also) and ground flax seeds. Note that flax seeds pass through your system virtually undigested unless ground into meal.

The next level of the pyramid is reserved for fish and seafood. Once again, not all fish and seafood are created equal in terms of the healthy fats or anti-inflammatory vitamins. Choose in particular the cold-water varieties of fish more often than not. Dr. Weil suggests 2-6 servings per week. A serving of fish is typically 4 oz. In some areas of the country, fish is seldom seen on the table because it is either not readily available or not affordable. It may therefore be less desirable and harder to integrate into the diet. In the recipes section, you will find the recipe for a delicious Mediterranean-style sauce that will appeal to the most hardened case of non-fish-eater you might imagine, with the possible exception of the Navajo nation of Native Americans. This population has no tradition of consuming fish, as they are a desert nation with no access to waters populated with native fish species. Assuming you are not of that nation, we will move on to the next level of the pyramid.

At this level, Dr. Weil has placed the class of whole soy foods, including soy milk, tempeh, tofu, edamame and soy nuts. We must caution that if you, like up to 10% of Americans, have thyroid disease whether diagnosed or not, soy products are contraindicated. If you are overweight, experience chronic tiredness, having thinning hair or eyebrows or other strong indications of hypothyroidism in particular, please see an endocrinologist before adding soy products to your diet. If you have been enjoying them with no problems, Dr. Weil suggests 1-2 servings a day.

Next on the pyramid is a level exclusively devoted to cooked Asian mushrooms. Dr. Weil, in other publications, cautions against consuming raw mushrooms or certain varieties of mushrooms because of their carcinogenic properties. However, lightly cooked button mushrooms makes the top 10 foods for vitamin D, so do not overlook this nutrient. Mushrooms seem to be one of those foods about which most people have a strong opinion; whether you love them or hate them, you at least are not indifferent to them. If you love them, try some new varieties to include the Asian ones. If you hate them, have you tried anything but the ubiquitous white button type? Why not try a couple more varieties to see whether you can learn to love them, or at least tolerate them for their beneficial properties? This is one of the few foods that you may enjoy in unlimited quantities based on Dr. Weil's recommendations.

We have now arrived at the level where this anti-inflammatory diet is going to turn many Americans on their heads with regard to changing eating habits. Other types of proteins than previously covered on lower levels come next. By this we mean lean meats, skinless poultry, eggs (preferably Omega-3 enriched), yogurt and high-quality natural cheeses. This entire class is suggested for 1-2 servings a week. Admittedly, most Americans would feel deprived if they got only 1-2 servings a day. But consider this: it is only since these foods became a relatively low-cost commodity that we have seen the drastic increase in the serious illnesses in which inflammation has been implicated. Could it be that our over-consumption of red meat and dairy has led directly to this trend? Consider also that the way we have been enjoying them in the most quantities since Col. Sanders and McDonald's became our go-to meals of convenience is precisely what leads to inflammation due to high bad-fat content. Now, could you possibly start to enjoy one extra meal per week of either fish or a vegetarian dish? Could you gradually increase that until you are consuming only 1-2 servings a week of this less-healthful form of protein? All right, we won't look that far ahead yet, but start with the baby step in order to get your diet under control.

After that blow, you will be glad to know that the next step on the pyramid allows you unlimited amounts—of healthy dried herbs and spices. Use them to make your simpler foods taste exciting and new; they're good for you! Next come supplements, which can be integrated into this diet to boost any nutrient you are having trouble getting enough of. Just take care that they are of high quality, in amounts not to exceed the recommended daily allowance, and approved by your medical advisors if you take any prescription medicine. Double check the informational material on all medicines and supplements even if your doctor does approve. Not all doctors have extensive knowledge of the interaction of supplements with prescription medication, and some supplements can render the medication ineffective. If you are currently taking prescription medications and would like to understand all interactions of supplements you might consider for their anti-oxidant effect, you can find several interaction checkers online by entering 'drug and supplement interaction checker' into your search engine. We would recommend selecting one from a reputable source, such as that provided by the Mayo Clinic.

The top two layers of the pyramid indicate a couple of items you might consider a treat, but also recommend you consume them sparingly. The next-to-top layer consists of red wines, with a suggested limit of 1-2 daily, although other recommendations limit this to 2-3 per week. The final layer is dark chocolate. Chocolate lovers love to shout from the rooftops that dark chocolate is healthy, and that is true to a certain extent. It is rich in antioxidants and contains what is considered healthy fat. However, because of its high fat content, it is also very high in calories, and frequently contains more sugar than is recommended, to counteract the bitter taste of pure chocolate. Consume this treat very sparingly, and choose the highest-quality that you can afford and the highest percentage of pure cocoa you can tolerate.

Although we have leaned heavily on Dr. Weil's recommendations, do not overlook the benefits of combining elements of the other similar diets, and do exercise your own judgment as regards how these nutrients are combined. US News & World Report has reviewed many of the popular published diets, including Dr. Weil's, and has some information about its conformity to accepted dietary guidelines; in summary, fat content is on the high end of the scale and a random daily menu from the book exceeds it; protein is on the low end of the scale, carbohydrates are under the recommended percent of daily calories, sodium exceeds it by 1/3-½, potassium was less than 1/3 the RDA, and vitamin D was not represented at all. Tracking the nutrients you get on a daily basis can be highly time-consuming, so when you select a published diet to follow, you may want to consider whether it meets accepted guidelines for key nutrients, and you may find that the reviews provided by US News & World Report helpful in doing so. As it turns out, the Mediterranean Diet meets more of the guidelines, although its primary purpose is weight reduction rather than anti-inflammatory.

In the end, it is up to you to do your due diligence or strike your own balance by choosing the most beneficial foods within your budget, taste and availability. If you do wish to follow a particular published diet and would like to see the review of it, search online using the name of the diet and adding US News at the end to lead you to the article. By the way, both of the diets we have compared lend themselves readily to special needs, such as kosher, low-sodium, vegetarian/vegan or gluten free. Both are also relatively easy to gradually incorporate into your lifestyle, as neither restricts an entire food or food group.

# Your Healthy Cholesterol Shopping List

The following table will assist you in shopping for a heart-healthy diet. You must be aware of other food restrictions you may have from unrelated conditions, such as gluten sensitivity or thyroid issues, and make adjustments accordingly. Most people should be able to find plenty of delicious, wholesome choices for healthy meal planning here.

## Foods to Eat in Plenty

These foods are good for you, filling, and will assist in raising HDL, lowering LDL, or both

### Fruits:

2-3 servings daily of a variety of fruits, including citrus fruits, berries, stone fruits like peaches and apricots, as well as tropical fruits. Top choice: blueberries, but all berries are good.

### Vegetables:

3-4 servings daily of a variety of vegetables, choosing from all available colors. Bell peppers of every color, carrots, green leafy vegetables — all vegetables are good.

### Foods with soluble fiber/whole grains:

Oatmeal, oat bran, barley, brown rice, quinoa, buckwheat, whole wheat if you do not have a gluten sensitivity.

### Legumes:

Lima beans, navy beans, kidney beans, pinto beans, lentils, chickpeas, hummus. We have left out soy because it has a minimal effect on blood cholesterol levels and a harmful effect on sensitive thyroid; however, if you like it and have no thyroid problems, it counts as a legume.

### Milk:

Almond or rice milk; soy milk if you can tolerate soy.

### Poultry:

Chicken and turkey, skin removed

### Fish:

At least three servings per week of cold-water, wild-caught fish varieties like salmon, herring, sardines, mackerel, tuna and trout. Beware of farmed fish. Broil, grill or steam your fish — frying them in oil cancels all benefit.

### Eggs:

Egg whites

### Desserts:

Sorbet, fresh fruit or fresh-frozen grapes and berries.

---

# Foods to Eat in Moderation

Many are high in calories, but contain nutrients that are beneficial.

### Oils:

Olive, Grapeseed, Flaxseed
Get more Omega-3 in your oil, and less Omega-6. An imbalance, which our Western diet promotes, leads to inflammation
Avocado-has been added here because although mostly fat and high in calories, just half an avocado a day for a few weeks can improve cholesterol levels and actually assist in weight loss.

### Starchy vegetables:

Potatoes except for sweet potatoes, corn (actually a grain, but often prepared as a vegetable)
Home-baked goods using whole grains and other healthy-choice List of Ingredients

### Nuts:

Especially almonds; nut butters. But beware of eating nuts that have been roasted in oil—raw is best.

### Dairy:

Skim or 1% milk, low-fat cheeses and cottage cheese, non-fat or low-fat yogurt, but beware of artificial sweeteners or lots of added sugar in the latter. Greek yogurt is a good choice - sweeten it with fruit and/or honey.

### Lean red meats, eggs.

Although the yolk of eggs has a lot of cholesterol, recent research shows it also contains substances that ameliorate the harmful effects. But choose low-cholesterol foods for the rest of the day on days you consume a whole egg.
Limit servings of meat, including the best choices, to two servings or 5 oz. per day.

### Dessert:

Dark chocolate, frozen yogurt

## Foods to Avoid

These foods have limited nutritional value, if any, and contain substances that tend to raise LDL.

Saturated and trans-fats: lard, butter, margarine, shortening and prepared foods with these List of Ingredients.
- French fries, other deep-fried vegetables
- Highly-processed foods: store-bought baked goods, sugary cereals, chips and many crackers
- Traditional re-fried beans
- Non-dairy creamer, whole milk and full-fat cheeses
- Processed meats: lunch meat, bacon, sausage, pate, foie gras
- Frozen entrees
- Oil-packed fish
- Shrimp and shellfish
- Whipped toppings, full-fat ice cream, cakes, pies, cookies

# Part 2 - Recipes To Keep Your Cholesterol Healthy

# Chicken Recipes

### Asian-Style Chicken Salad

Serving 4
**List of Ingredients**
4 cups (1 L) water

1 brown onion, halved

2 single chicken breast fillets

1 carrot, peeled, cut into matchsticks

5.30 oz (150g) snow peas, trimmed, thinly sliced

1 red capsicum, deseeded, thinly sliced

1/2 wombok (Chinese cabbage), hard core removed, finely shredded

3 green shallots, ends trimmed, thinly sliced diagonally

1/2 cup fresh coriander leaves

2 tbs fresh lime juice

1 tbs fish sauce

2 tsp brown sugar

1 fresh red chili, deseeded, chopped

**Preparation**

Place water, onion and chicken in a saucepan over medium heat. Bring to the boil. Reduce heat to low and cook, covered, for 10 minutes or until cooked. Drain chicken and discard onion.

Place carrot and snow peas in a bowl. Cover with boiling water. Set aside for 1 minute or until bright green and tender crisp. Refresh under cold running water.

Shred chicken. Place chicken, carrot, snow peas, capsicum, wombok, shallot and coriander in a bowl. Combine lime juice, fish sauce, sugar and chili in a jar. Pour over salad and combine. Divide among serving bowls to serve.

## Chicken -Sweet Potato - Chickpeas

Serving 4
**List of Ingredients**
2 red onions, halved, cut into thick wedges
21.20 oz (600g) sweet potato (kumara), peeled, cut into 3cm pieces
4 tomatoes, halved
2 garlic cloves, thinly sliced
2 tbs olive oil
8 (about 21.90 oz or 620g) chicken thigh fillets
8.50 oz (240g) can chickpeas, rinsed, and drained
1/4 cup chopped fresh continental parsley
**Preparation**
Preheat oven to 428.00°F (220°C). Combine the onion, sweet potato, tomato, garlic and half the oil in a bowl. Transfer to large baking tray. Bake for 15 minutes.
Meanwhile, heat remaining oil in a large frying pan. Season the chicken with salt and pepper. Cook for 1-2 minutes each side or until golden.
Add the chicken to the tray and bake for a further 10 minutes or until the chicken is cooked through. Add chickpeas and parsley. Toss until heated through.

## Chicken Lentil Spinach

Serving 4
**List of Ingredients**
1 1/2 tbs olive oil

4 x 6 oz (170g) chicken breast fillets, cut into 3cm cubes

1 red onion, finely chopped

1 celery stalk, finely chopped, plus 1 tbs chopped celery leaves

2 garlic cloves, finely chopped

2 tsp chopped thyme leaves

250ml (1 cup) salt-reduced chicken stock

4.20 oz (120g) baby spinach leaves

2 x 14.10 oz (400g) cans brown lentils, rinsed, drained

4 crusty bread rolls, to serve

**Preparation**
Heat oil in a deep fry pan over medium-high heat. In 2 batches, add chicken and brown all over for 3-4 minutes. Remove from the pan and set aside.

Reduce heat to medium, add onion, celery stalk, garlic and thyme, then season. Cook for 5 minutes, stirring, until vegetables soften. Return chicken to pan with stock, bring to the boil, then cover and simmer over low heat for 10 minutes or until chicken is cooked.

Stir in spinach, celery leaves and lentils, then cook for 3-4 minutes until spinach is wilted and lentils are warmed through. Serve with crusty bread.

## Moroccan Chicken Carrot and Chickpea

Serving 4

**List of Ingredients**

2 bunches baby (Dutch) carrots, trimmed, scrubbed

1 1/2 tbs olive oil

4 x 6 oz (170g) skinless chicken breast fillets

1 tbs sumac (see note)

2 tbs white wine vinegar

1 garlic clove, crushed

1 tsp honey

2 x 14.10 oz (400g) cans chickpeas, rinsed, drained

1/2 cup (80g) sunflower seeds, toasted

1 cup flat-leaf parsley leaves

**Preparation**

Preheat the oven to 356.00°F (180°C). Spread the carrots on a baking tray in a single layer. Season, then drizzle over 1 tbs oil and 2 tbs water. Roast for 10-12 minutes until the carrots soften slightly.

Meanwhile, lightly oil a chargrill pan with the remaining olive oil. Heat over medium-high heat. Season the chicken with sea salt and freshly ground black pepper and rub with the sumac. Cook for 3-4 minutes each side until browned. Remove the tray from the oven, turn the carrots then place the chicken on top. Roast for a further 10-12 minutes until the chicken is cooked through.

Whisk the vinegar, garlic and honey together in a large bowl. Season, then add chickpeas, sunflower seeds, parsley and carrots and toss to combine. Divide salad among plates, then top with the chicken.

# Chicken Chickpea Tabouli Salad

Serving 4
**List of Ingredients**
1/2 cup (90g) burghul

1 cup (250ml) boiling water

2 tsp olive oil

3 (about 21.20 oz or 600g) single chicken breast fillets, excess fat trimmed

1 x 14.10 oz (400g) can chickpeas, rinsed, drained

1 bunch fresh mint, leaves picked, coarsely chopped

1 bunch fresh continental parsley, leaves picked, coarsely chopped

3 ripe tomatoes, coarsely chopped

4 green shallots, ends trimmed, thinly sliced

1/2 cup (125ml) fresh lemon juice

Lebanese bread, to serve

**Preparation**

Place the burghul in a heatproof bowl. Pour over the boiling water and set aside for 12 minutes or until soft. Drain and transfer to a large bowl.

Meanwhile, heat the oil in a non-stick frying pan over medium-high heat. Add chicken and cook for 4-5 minutes each side or until cooked. Thickly slice.

Add the chicken, chickpeas, mint, parsley, tomato and shallot to the burghul and combine.

Add lemon juice and season with salt and pepper. Toss to combine. Arrange on a serving platter and serve with Lebanese bread.

# Chicken Mango Salad with Walnuts

Serving 4

**List of Ingredients**

4 (about 4.40 oz or 125g each) single chicken breast fillets, excess fat trimmed

1/2 tsp olive oil

1 Calypso mango

1 x 400g pkt fresh complete salad mix

2 Lebanese cucumbers, coarsely chopped

3.50 oz (100g) snow peas, trimmed, thinly sliced lengthways

1/4 cup (30g) walnuts, coarsely chopped

1/4 cup (60ml) fat-free French dressing

4 pieces whole meal Lebanese bread, halved

**Preparation**

Preheat a barbecue flat plate or chargrill on medium-high. Brush both sides of the chicken evenly with the oil. Season with pepper. Add the chicken to the flat plate or grill and reduce heat to medium. Cook for 4 minutes each side or until cooked through. Transfer to a plate. Cover with foil and set aside for 5 minutes to rest.

Meanwhile, use a small sharp knife to cut down either side of the mango seed to remove the cheeks. Peel and cut the flesh into thin strips. Combine the mango, salad mix, cucumber, snow peas and walnuts in a large bowl. Add the French dressing and toss until well combined.

Thinly slice the chicken across the grain. Divide the salad among serving bowls and top with the chicken. Season with salt and pepper. Serve immediately with bread, if desired.

# Snow Pea Pumpkin Chicken Salad

Serving 4
**List of Ingredients**
5 cups (1.25L) cold water

1 brown onion, peeled, halved

2 sprigs fresh continental parsley

6 black peppercorns

Pinch of salt

2 (7.10 oz or 200g each) single chicken breast fillets

26.50 oz (750g) butternut pumpkin, peeled, deseeded, cut into 2cm pieces

Olive oil spray

2 tsp sesame seeds

7.10 oz (200g) snow peas, trimmed, halved diagonally

3.50 oz (100g) baby spinach leaves

Balsamic vinegar, to serve

**Preparation**

Place the water, onion, parsley, peppercorns and salt in a saucepan. Bring to the boil over medium heat. Add the chicken and cover with a lid. Remove from heat and set aside for 30 minutes to poach. Use a slotted spoon to remove chicken from the poaching liquid and set aside to cool slightly. Discard the liquid.

Preheat oven to 392.00°F (200°C). Line a large baking tray with non-stick baking paper. Place the pumpkin on the lined tray. Spray with olive oil spray and season with pepper. Roast in oven, turning once halfway through cooking, for 30 minutes or until golden.

Meanwhile, place the sesame seeds in a small frying pan over medium heat. Cook, stirring, for 4-5 minutes or until toasted.

Bring a medium saucepan of water to the boil. Add the snow peas and cook for 1-2 minutes or until bright green and tender crisp. Rinse under cold running water. Drain.

Use your fingers to shred the chicken. Combine chicken, pumpkin, snow peas and spinach in a large bowl. Divide evenly among the serving plates. Drizzle over the balsamic vinegar and sprinkle with the toasted sesame seeds. Serve immediately.

# Indian-Spiced Quinoa with Chicken

Serving 4

**List of Ingredients**

2 tbs peanut oil
1 tbs black mustard seeds
12 fresh curry leaves*, plus extra to garnish
2 tsp garam masala*
3 long green chilies, seeds removed, thinly sliced
1 large onion, coarsely grated
1 1/2 cups (200g) quinoa
1/2 cup (110g) green split peas
3 cups (750ml) salt-reduced chicken stock
1 1/2 cups shredded cooked chicken
2.80 oz (80g) baby spinach leaves, roughly shredded

**Preparation**

Heat oil in a large pan over medium heat. Add mustard seeds and cook until they begin to pop. Add curry leaves, garam masala, chili and onion, and cook until onion is golden and spices are aromatic. Add quinoa and peas, and stir to coat in spice mixture. Add stock and 1 cup (250ml) boiling water. Simmer over low heat for 25 minutes, then add chicken and spinach and heat through for 5 minutes. Season to taste and serve garnished with extra curry leaves.

## Lime Coriander Spinach Chicken

Serving 4
**List of Ingredients**
2 fresh coriander roots

2 garlic cloves

1 tbs olive oil

1/2 cup (125ml) lime juice

4 x 6.40 oz (180g) skinless chicken breast fillets

3 bunches English spinach, trimmed

1/3 cup slivered almonds, toasted

1/3 cup sultanas

1/2 tsp cinnamon

**Preparation**
Use a mortar and pestle to pound coriander and garlic with a little sea salt. Add oil and 1/3 cup (80ml) lime juice and stir to combine. Place chicken in a bowl, pour marinade over, cover and refrigerate for 15-20 minutes.
Preheat and lightly oil a chargrill or barbecue to medium-high. Cook chicken for about 5 minutes each side, or until cooked through.

Meanwhile, cook spinach in a steamer for 1 minute until just wilted. Transfer to a bowl and toss with almonds, sultanas, cinnamon and remaining lime juice.

Season with salt and pepper. Serve chicken on a bed of spinach.

## Lime Pearl Barley Corn Salad Chicken

Serving 4
**List of Ingredients**
1/4 cup (60ml) fresh lime juice

2 tsp paprika

1 garlic clove, crushed

2 x 7.10 oz (200g) single chicken breast fillets

1 cup (220g) pearl barley

Olive oil spray

1 1/2 cups (285g) fresh corn kernels

1 small red capsicum, halved, deseeded, finely chopped

4 shallots, ends trimmed, thinly sliced

1/2 cup fresh continental parsley leaves

**Preparation**
Combine the lime juice, paprika and garlic in a jug. Place the chicken in a shallow glass or ceramic dish. Add half the lime juice mixture to the chicken and turn to coat. Cover with plastic wrap and place in the fridge for 20 minutes to marinate.

Meanwhile, cook the barley in a large saucepan of boiling water for 20 minutes or until tender. Rinse under cold running water. Drain. Transfer to a large bowl.

Heat a non-stick frying pan over high heat. Spray with olive oil spray. Add the corn and cook, stirring occasionally, for 2 minutes. Add the capsicum and shallot and cook, stirring, for 1 minute or until the corn is light golden. Add the corn mixture, parsley and remaining lime juice mixture to the barley. Taste and season with pepper. Stir until well combined.

Wipe the pan clean with paper towel. Place over medium-high heat. Spray with olive oil spray. Drain the chicken from the marinade. Cook for 4 minutes each side or until cooked through. Set aside to cool slightly.

Thinly slice the chicken. Divide the barley mixture among serving bowls. Top with the chicken to serve.

## Chicken Wheat Salad

Serving 4
**List of Ingredients**
2 tbs fresh lemon juice

2 tsp honey

3 tsp sumac

17.60 oz (500g) single chicken breast fillets

2 tsp olive oil

1 cup (170g) burghul (cracked wheat)

7.10 oz (200g) flat beans, topped, cut into 3cm lengths

1/2 cup fresh continental parsley leaves

1/3 cup (50g) sweetened dried cranberries

2 tbs toasted pine nuts

Olive oil spray

**Preparation**

Combine half the lemon juice, half the honey and 2 teaspoons of the sumac in a shallow glass or ceramic dish. Add the chicken and turn to coat. Cover with plastic wrap and place in the fridge for 20 minutes to marinate. Whisk together the oil and the remaining lemon juice, honey and sumac in a small jug.

Meanwhile, place the burghul in a heatproof bowl. Cover with boiling water. Set aside for 20 minutes to soak. Strain through a fine sieve and use the back of a spoon to press out excess water. Transfer to a bowl.

Preheat oven to 374.00°F (190°C). Cook the beans in a saucepan of boiling water for 3-4 minutes or until bright green and tender crisp. Refresh under cold running water. Drain. Add the beans, parsley, cranberries and pine nuts to the burghul and toss to combine.

Heat a frying pan over high heat. Spray lightly with olive oil spray. Drain the chicken from the marinade. Add the chicken to the pan and cook for 2 minutes each side or until golden brown. Transfer to a baking tray and bake in oven for 10-12 minutes or until cooked through. Set aside for 2 minutes to rest. Thinly slice across the grain. Divide the salad among serving plates. Top with the chicken and drizzle over the dressing to serve.

## Chicken Pasta Salad

Serving 2
**List of Ingredients**
5.30 oz (150g) dried farfalle pasta

1/4 cup (40g) frozen green peas, thawed

1/4 barbecued chicken (breast section)

1 small carrot, peeled, coarsely grated

10 cherry tomatoes, halved

2 tbs chopped fresh continental parsley

**Dressing**
3 tsp extra virgin olive oil

1 tbs white wine vinegar

1/2 tsp Dijon mustard

Salt & freshly ground black pepper

**Preparation**
Cook the pasta in a large saucepan of salted boiling water following packet directions until al dente. Add the peas in the last 2 minutes of cooking. Drain. Refresh under cold running water and drain well.

Remove the chicken meat from the bones. Discard the bones and skin. Shred the chicken and place in a bowl with the cooked pasta and peas. Add the carrot, tomato and parsley, and gently toss until combined.

To make the dressing, combine the oil, vinegar and mustard in a screw-top jar. Season with salt and pepper and shake until well combined. Pour dressing over pasta salad and gently toss to combine. Store salad in an airtight container.

## Delicious Chicken Tortilla

**List of Ingredients**
1 sliced chicken breast
1 tsp olive oil
1 finely chopped onion
1 roughly chopped red or green pepper
A few small tortillas
1 peeled and grated carrot
1 cup of lettuce
14 oz. drained kidney beans
1 tbsp crème fraiche
Salt and pepper

**Preparation**
Fry the onion and pepper in the tsp of olive oil for approximately 2 minutes.
Add the chicken pieces and continue frying until the chicken is cooked and nicely browned.
In a separate bowl combine and crème fraiche and kidney beans and mash.
Spread the mixture onto a few tortillas and then add the chicken, lettuce leaves and carrots before you roll it up.
Guaranteed to be delicious!

# Thai Chicken Noodle Salad

**List of Ingredients**
2 chopped chicken breasts
2 chopped cloves of garlic
1 lime (use juice and zest)
1 tsp oil
2 tbsp chopped coriander
1 orange (use juice and zest)
¼ cucumber sliced
½ chopped red chili
3 oz. halved blanched beans
1 cup cooked noodles
3 sliced spring onions
I tsp honey

**Preparation**
Place the chicken in a medium sized dish and cover with the juice and zest from the lime. Place in the refrigerator and leave to marinate for approximately 30 min.

Place the tsp of olive oil in a frying pan and fry the garlic and chicken until the chicken is properly cooked (should take about 8 min).

In a large bowl combine the onion, coriander, beans, cucumber, noodles and chili.

Make a dressing out of the honey and orange and drizzle over salad

To serve, place salad in plates and finish off by placing the fried chicken on top.

## Sweet and Sour Chicken Salad

**List of Ingredients**
4 large chicken breasts (boneless and skinless)
Teriyaki sauce (enough to marinate chicken in)
8 won tons
1 head lettuce chopped
2 tbsp + 2 tsp vinegar
3 tbsp + 2 tsp canola oil
¾ tsp paprika
Ground black pepper
1 tbsp sweet and sour sauce
1 tbsp sesame seeds (toasted)
1 tsp salt
¼ cup green onions

**Preparation**
Marinate chicken pieces in Teriyaki sauce for a few hours before baking or placing in microwave until cooked through. Cut into cubes.
Fry won ton in 1 tbsp canola oil and drain.
Combine the vinegar, remaining canola oil, paprika, black pepper, sweet and sour sauce and salt in a pot and bring to a boil. Once boiling starts turn off heat and allow to cool.
In a salad bowl combine the lettuce, chicken, sesame seeds, and green onions.
Just before serving add the dressing and won tons and your sticky delicious salad is ready!

## Chicken and Berry Salad

**List of Ingredients**
1 cup chicken strips
1 cup blueberries
1 cup finely grated carrots
1 medium sized bag crisp lettuce
1 tsp canola oil
1 tsp cayenne pepper
1/2 tsp ginger
1/2 cup raspberries

**Preparation**
Combine the cayenne pepper and ginger and spice chicken strips before cooking in a pan for approximately 5 minutes. In a large salad bowl combine the lettuce, carrots, blueberries, raspberries and cooked chicken strips. Drizzle with any fat free dressing and add salt and pepper to taste.

# Chicken, Red Pepper and Avocado Focaccia

**List of Ingredients**

18 inch focaccia
1/2 cup roasted red sweet peppers, sliced
4 thick slices roast chicken (cooked)
1/3 cup light mayonnaise
1/3 cup mashed avocado

**Preparation**

Cut focaccia in half and spread both sides with low fat mayonnaise.

Top with roast chicken slices, red peppers and mashed avocado. Simple yet delicious.

# Grilled Chicken Breasts – Mediterranean Style

**List of Ingredients**
4 large chicken breasts
1 tsp oregano leaves
2 tbsp grated lemon peel
1 chopped red onion
20 kalamata olives (pitted)
4 Roma tomatoes (plum) quartered
1/2 cup low fat feta cheese (preferably tomato and basil flavoured)

**Preparation**
Cut 4 large pieces of heavy duty foil that you will be using for grilling the chicken (18 by 12 inch). Preheat Grill.

Lay out the sheets of foil and on each one place a chicken breast, slices of tomato, a tbsp of chopped onion, and 5 olives. Once that is done top each chicken breast with ¼ cup of the feta cheese.

Now wrap up each chicken breast in the foil by pulling the sides over. Seal on all sides in preparation for grilling.

Place the packages on the grill over medium heat and allow to cool for approximately 25 minutes, turning halfway through the cooking time (after about 12 minutes).

Guaranteed to be tender and delicious!

## Thai Chicken Stir Fry

**List of Ingredients**
14 oz. sliced chicken breast fillets
11/2 cups doongara rice
3 cups water
1 tsp sesame oil
1/4 cup soy sauce (reduced salt)
1/4 cup lime juice
1 cup fresh baby corn
1/4 cup water (extra)
2 tbsp honey
2 chopped red Thai chilies
2 tsp corn flour
2 tsp lime rind, finely grated
3 cups bean sprouts
2 cups fresh Thai basil leaves
1 cup fresh coriander
1 tbsp peanut oil
3 cloves garlic, crushed
2 finely sliced red onions

**Preparation**
To make a marinade, combine honey, chili, sesame oil, cornflour, juice and sauce in bowl. Place chicken in mixture and coat completely. Cover and place in fridge for at least an hour.

Cook rice according to package instructions.

Remove chicken from marinade. Keep marinade

Brown the chicken in a wok, in batches using 1/2 of the peanut oil. Remove from wok and place to one side. Using the rest of the peanut oil fry the onion, garlic, corn and tender, but not overcooked. Place browned chicken back into the wok with the leftover marinade, extra water and rind. Keep frying until the chicken is cooked through.
Before serving sprinkle with herbs and sprouts. Serve delicious chicken and veggie mix with rice.

# Fish Recipes

## Fish & Vegetables

Serving 4
**List of Ingredients**
2 zucchinis, cut into wedges

2 red onions, cut into wedges

3 tomatoes, cut into wedges

1/4 cup pitted black olives

1/4 cup (60ml) olive oil

4 x 6.30 oz (180g) thick skinless white fish fillets (such as ling)

1 small garlic clove, crushed

1 tbs lemon juice

1 tbs Dijon mustard

1/2 cup roughly chopped flat-leaf parsley

**Preparation**
Preheat the oven to 392.00°F (200°C).

Toss the zucchini, onion, tomato and olives with 1 tablespoon of the oil in a baking dish. Brush another tablespoon of oil over the fish and place on the vegetables. Place in the oven and bake for 25-30 minutes until cooked through.

Whisk together the garlic, lemon juice, mustard and remaining oil to make a dressing.

Divide the cooked vegetables among plates and top each with a piece of fish.

Drizzle the fish with the dressing and scatter with chopped parsley.

## Mediterranean Baked Fish

Serves 4
**List of Ingredients**
2 tsp olive oil
1 large onion, sliced
1 can diced tomatoes, with juice
1 bay leaf
1 clove garlic, minced
¾ C apple juice
¼ C lemon juice
¼ C orange juice
1 T freshly grated orange zest
1 tsp fennel seeds, crushed
1 ½ tsp Italian seasonings (or ½ tsp each ground oregano, thyme, basil)
Black pepper to taste
1 lb. fish fillets
**Preparation**
In large non-stick skillet, heat oil; add onion and sauté until soft. Add remaining list of ingredients, crushing the tomatoes a little with your spoon or fork; stir occasionally while simmering an additional 30 minutes, uncovered. Arrange fish in a shallow baking dish, cover with sauce. Bake uncovered about 15 minutes or until fish flakes easily. Alternatively, grill fish to taste and serve sauce on the side.

## Fish Fennel Tomato Oregano

Serving 4
**List of Ingredients**
17.60 oz (500g) Baby Coliban (Chat) potatoes (see note)

2 large fennel bulbs, trimmed, cut into thin wedges

2 tsp olive oil

1 x 8.80 oz (250g) punnet cherry tomatoes, halved

1 tbs balsamic glaze

4 (about 4.40 oz or 125g each) white fish fillets

2 tbs fresh oregano leaves

**Preparation**
Preheat oven to 392.00ºF (200°C). Prick potatoes with a fork all over. Place on paper towel in microwave. Cook on High/800watts/100% for 5 minutes. Cool slightly. Halve. Place the potato and fennel on a large baking tray. Drizzle over the oil. Season with pepper. Bake for 25-30 minutes or until potato starts to turn golden. Add the tomato. Drizzle over the balsamic glaze. Bake for 5 minutes.
Place fish on top of the potato mixture. Sprinkle with half the oregano. Bake for a further 8-10 minutes or until fish flakes when tested with a fork in thickest part.

Divide the potato, fennel, tomato and fish among serving plates. Drizzle over the juices from the tray. Sprinkle with remaining oregano to serve.

# Salmon Potato Bean Salad

Serving 4

**List of Ingredients**

4 (about 6.40 oz or 180g each) salmon fillets
12 chat (small coliban) potatoes, halved
1 tbs extra virgin olive oil
1 tbs white wine vinegar
7.10 oz (200g) green beans, topped, halved
1 x 8.80 oz (250g) cherry tomatoes, halved
2.10 oz (60g) baby spinach leaves
1 tbs drained capers
Freshly ground black pepper
Lemon wedges

**Preparation**

Preheat oven to 356.00ºF (180°C). Cut four 40cm-diameter discs from non-stick baking paper. Place 1 salmon fillet on 1 half of each paper disc. Fold the discs in half to enclose the salmon. Fold over the edges to seal the parcels. Place the parcels on 2 baking trays. Bake in preheated oven, swapping trays halfway through cooking, for 10-12 minutes or until parcels puff and salmon flakes when tested with a fork. Remove from oven.

Meanwhile, cook the potato in a large saucepan of boiling water for 15 minutes or until tender. Drain well. Place in a large heatproof bowl. Place the oil and vinegar in a screw-top jar and shake until well combined. Drizzle the potato with dressing and gently toss to coat.

Place the beans in a large heatproof bowl and cover with boiling water. Set aside for 3 minutes or until bright green and tender crisp. Drain well. Add the beans to the potato mixture along with the tomato, spinach and capers, and gently toss to combine. Divide the salad among serving plates. Top with the salmon and season with pepper. Serve immediately with lemon wedges.

# Salmon Fennel Orange Chickpeas

Serving 4
**List of Ingredients**
2 oranges, peeled

1 fennel bulb, trimmed, very thinly sliced

1 x 14.10 oz (400g) can Edgell Salt-Reduced Chickpeas, rinsed, drained

1/2 red onion, thinly sliced

1/3 cup fresh continental parsley leaves

2 tbs chopped fresh dill

1 large (about 13.20 oz or 375g) skinless salmon fillet, pin boned

Olive oil spray

50g baby rocket leaves

Lemon wedges, to serve

**Preparation**
Holding 1 orange over a large bowl to catch any juice, use a sharp knife to cut along either side of the white membrane to remove the segments. Add to the bowl. Use your hands to squeeze the juice from the remaining flesh. Repeat with remaining orange.

Add the fennel, chickpeas, onion, parsley and dill to the bowl. Season with pepper. Toss to combine.

Preheat a barbecue flat plate or chargrill on high. Cut salmon lengthways into 8 slices. Spray lightly with olive oil spray and season with pepper. Cook on barbecue for 1 minute each side for medium or until cooked to your liking. Flake into bite-sized pieces. Add salmon and rocket to the orange mixture and toss to combine. Divide among serving dishes and serve with lemon wedges.

## Harissa Fish

Serving 4
**List of Ingredients**
1 1/2 tablespoons harissa

4 x 7.10 oz (200g) blue-eye fillets, skin removed

1 red capsicum, cut into quarters, deseeded

2 x 14.10 oz (400g) cans chickpeas, drained, rinsed

1/2 cup flat-leaf parsley leaves

4 green onions, thinly sliced

1 lemon, juiced

Olive oil cooking spray

1/3 cup low-fat natural yoghurt

**Preparation**
Combine harissa and 1/2 cup cold water in a shallow ceramic dish. Add fish fillets and turn to coat. Cover and refrigerate for 30 minutes, if time permits.
Preheat a barbecue grill on high heat. Place capsicum, skin side down, on grill. Cook for 8 to 10 minutes or until skin turns black. Transfer capsicum to a plastic bag. Twist top to seal and stand for 5 minutes. Peel and discard skin. Roughly chop capsicum and place in a bowl.

Add chickpeas, parsley and green onions to capsicum. Drizzle over 2 tablespoons lemon juice. Toss gently to combine.

Reduce barbecue grill to medium heat. Spray both sides of fish with oil. Cook for 3 minutes each side or until cooked through. Place fish and salad on plates. Top with yoghurt. Season with pepper and serve.

# Citrus Fish Salad

Serving 4

**List of Ingredients**

1 tbs olive oil

21.20 oz (600g) skinless flathead fillets

2 tbs red wine vinegar

Finely grated zest and juice of 1 lemon

Finely grated zest and juice of 1/2 orange

1 tsp Dijon mustard

2.80 oz (80g) baby frisee (curly endive) or other baby salad leaves (see note)

1 cup flat-leaf parsley leaves

1 red onion, thinly sliced

2 tbs drained baby capers

4 slices dark rye bread, toasted, torn

**Preparation**

Heat 2 tsp oil in a large non-stick pan over medium-high heat. Add fish, season, and cook for 2 minutes or until golden. Turn fish, then add vinegar and 1 cup (250ml) hot water. Bring to a simmer and cook for 2 minutes or until cooked through. Transfer to a plate using a slotted spoon. Combine remaining oil, zests, juices and mustard in a large bowl. Season to taste. Add remaining list of ingredients and flake fish over. Toss gently to combine, then serve.

## Fish Stew

Serving 4

**List of Ingredients**

1 tablespoon extra-light olive oil

4 garlic cloves, finely chopped

1 teaspoon ground turmeric

2 x 14.10 oz (400g) cans whole peeled tomatoes

14.10 oz (400g) can cannellini beans, drained, rinsed

21.20 oz (600g) ling fillets, cut into large pieces (see note)

1/3 cup fresh coriander leaves, chopped

4 crusty wholegrain bread rolls, to serve

**Preparation**

Heat oil in a large saucepan over medium heat. Add garlic. Cook, stirring, for 1 minute. Add turmeric. Cook, stirring, for 30 seconds. Reduce heat to low. Stir in tomatoes and 1 cup of cold water. Cover and bring to the boil. Simmer, covered, for 10 minutes.

Add beans and return to the boil. Add fish. Cover and cook for 5 minutes or until fish is cooked through.

Spoon stew into bowls and sprinkle with coriander. Serve with bread rolls.

## Fish Chili Chickpea Salad

Serving 4
**List of Ingredients**
2 tsp olive oil

4 shallots, trimmed, thinly sliced

2 tsp grated fresh ginger

2 garlic cloves, crushed

2 long fresh green chilies, seeded, thinly sliced

2 x 14.10 oz (400g) cans no-added-salt chickpeas, rinsed, drained

1 1/2 tbs fresh lemon juice

1 tsp ground sumac

7.10 oz (200g) green round beans, topped, cut into 3cm lengths

1/3 cup (50g) reduced-fat feta, crumbled

3 celery sticks, trimmed, cut into matchsticks

1/3 cup fresh continental parsley leaves

4 (about 5.30 oz or 150g each) white fish fillets

## Preparation

Heat half the oil in a large non-stick frying pan over medium heat. Cook the shallot, ginger, garlic and chili, stirring, for 2 minutes or until aromatic. Stir in the chickpeas, lemon juice and half the sumac.

Cook the beans in a saucepan of boiling water for 2 minutes or until bright green and tender crisp. Drain. Add the beans, feta, celery and parsley to the chickpea mixture and stir to combine. Season with pepper.

Heat a large non-stick frying pan over high heat. Brush the fish with the remaining oil. Cook for 3 minutes. Turn and cook for 1 minute or until just cooked through.

Divide the salad among serving plates. Top with the fish and sprinkle with the remaining sumac.

## Fish Chickpea Puree

Serving 4
**List of Ingredients**
1 tablespoon olive oil
1 brown onion, finely chopped
1 garlic clove, crushed
1 1/2 teaspoons ground cumin
1 cup reduced-salt chicken stock
2 x 14.80 oz (420g) cans chickpeas, drained, rinsed
1 tablespoon lemon juice
1/2 cup parsley, roughly chopped
4 pieces fish fillets (such as mullet, redfish or silver trevally)
2 cups baby spinach
2 tomatoes, chopped
**Preparation**
Heat a saucepan over medium heat until hot. Add 2 teaspoons of oil, onion, garlic and cumin. Cook, stirring, for 3 to 5 minutes or until soft. Add stock and chickpeas. Bring to the boil. Reduce heat to low. Simmer for 10 minutes. Remove from heat. Stir in lemon juice. Process or blend until smooth. Stir in parsley, and pepper.

Meanwhile, heat a non-stick frying pan or chargrill over medium heat. Brush fish with remaining 2 teaspoons of oil. Season lightly with pepper. Cook for 3 to 5 minutes each side or until just cooked through.

Spoon warm chickpea puree onto 4 serving plates. Top with baby spinach, fish and chopped tomatoes. Serve.

## Fish Casserole

Serving 4
**List of Ingredients**
Olive oil cooking spray

1 brown onion, halved, thinly sliced

12.40 oz (350g) orange sweet potato, peeled, cut into 2cm pieces

2 small zucchini, cut into 1cm pieces

7.10 oz (200g) broccoli, trimmed, cut into florets

1 small (8.80 oz or 250g) eggplant, diced

28.20 oz (800g) can diced tomatoes

1/3 cup fresh oregano leaves

17.60 oz (500g) white fish fillets, cut into large pieces

1 small white bread stick, sliced, toasted

**Preparation**
Heat a heavy-based saucepan over medium heat. Lightly spray with oil. Add onion and cook, stirring, for 2 minutes or until golden.

Add sweet potato. Cook, stirring, for 3 minutes. Add zucchini, broccoli, eggplant, tomatoes and 1/4 cup oregano. Bring to boil.

Reduce heat to low. Cover and cook for 8 to 10 minutes or until sweet potato is tender. Stir in fish. Simmer, uncovered, for 4 to 5 minutes or until fish is cooked through.

Sprinkle with remaining oregano. Serve casserole with toasted bread.

## Chili Fish Ginger

Serving 4
**List of Ingredients**
1 1/4 cups (250g) long-grain rice

Canola oil spray

4 (about 5.30 oz or 150g each) white fish fillets

2 tbs sushi seasoning

2 tbs salt-reduced soy sauce

5cm-piece fresh ginger, peeled, cut into matchsticks

1 long red chili, seeded, thinly sliced

7.10 oz (200g) snow peas, halved diagonally lengthways

1 bunch choy sum, trimmed, leaves separated

2 tbs chopped fresh coriander

2 tbs chopped fresh mint

Fresh mint leaves, to serve

## Preparation

Cook rice following packet directions. Meanwhile, heat a large non-stick frying pan over medium-high heat. Spray with oil. Cook fish for 2-3 minutes each side or until cooked through. Transfer to a plate. Add sushi seasoning, soy sauce, ginger and chili to pan. Cook for 1 minute or until mixture is heated through and slightly reduced.

Meanwhile, cook snow peas and choy sum in a saucepan of boiling water until bright green and tender-crisp. Drain. Add coriander and chopped mint to rice and stir to combine. Top with mint leaves.

Divide snow peas, choy sum and fish among plates. Drizzle with ginger mixture and serve with rice.

## Herb-Crusted Fish and Crushed Carrots

Serving 4
**List of Ingredients**
Olive oil, to grease

3 slices white bread, crusts removed, coarsely torn

2 tbs chopped fresh continental parsley

1 tbs chopped fresh chives

2 tsp chopped fresh tarragon

1 tsp chopped fresh dill

4 (about 7.10 oz or 200g each) firm white fish fillets (such as blue-eye trevalla)

21.20 oz (600g) carrots, peeled, coarsely chopped

1 bunch broccolini, ends trimmed

3.50 oz (100g) green beans, topped

1 tbs extra virgin olive oil

**Preparation**

Preheat oven to 392.00ºF (200°C). Brush a baking tray with olive oil to lightly grease. Place the bread, parsley, chives, tarragon and dill in the bowl of a food processor and process until finely chopped. Transfer to a large plate.

Press both sides of the fish into the parsley mixture to coat. Place on the prepared tray. Bake for 12 minutes or until the fish flakes easily when tested with a fork in the thickest part.

Meanwhile, cook the carrot in a saucepan of boiling water for 10 minutes or until tender. Use a slotted spoon to transfer to a heatproof bowl. Add the broccolini and beans to the pan and cook for 1 minute or until bright green and tender crisp. Drain.

Use a fork to coarsely mash the carrot. Divide the carrot, broccolini and beans among serving plates. Top with the fish. Drizzle over the extra virgin olive oil to serve.

## Orange Trout Salad

Serving 4
**List of Ingredients**
4 (6.40 oz or 180g each) ocean trout fillets, skin removed

2 tablespoons dijon mustard

1 tablespoon honey

2 large oranges

1 tablespoon apple cider vinegar

2 teaspoons olive oil

2.80 oz (80g) rocket

1/2 cup pitted kalamata olives

**Preparation**
Preheat grill on high heat. Line a baking tray with baking paper. Place fish on tray. Whisk mustard and honey together in a bowl. Reserve 1 tablespoon of mixture. Brush trout with remaining mustard mixture. Cook under grill for 5 to 7 minutes or until light golden and just cooked through. Remove to a plate. Cover with foil to keep warm.

Meanwhile, peel and segment oranges over a bowl, reserving 1 tablespoon of juice. Whisk reserved juice, vinegar, oil and reserved mustard mixture together in a bowl.

Combine rocket, olives, orange segments and dressing in a bowl. Serve fish with rocket and orange salad.

## Moroccan Salmon

Serving 4
**List of Ingredients**
3 garlic cloves, crushed

1/4 cup (30g) cumin seeds

1/4 cup (25g) coriander seeds

11/2 tbs sweet paprika

11/2 tbs finely grated lemon rind

4 (about 8.10 oz or 230g each) salmon fillets

Olive oil spray

Lemon wedges, to serve

**Mint & lemon salad**
1/2 cup (90g) burghul

1 cup (250ml) boiling water

1 tbs finely grated lemon rind

1/2 cup (125ml) fresh lemon juice

1 x 14.10 oz (400g) can chickpeas, rinsed, drained

1 bunch fresh mint, chopped

1 bunch fresh chives, chopped

**Preparation**

Place garlic, cumin, coriander, paprika and lemon rind in a mortar and crush with a pestle to form a paste. Rub over both sides of salmon. Cover and place in fridge for 3 hours to marinate.

Meanwhile, to make the salad, place the burghul in a bowl. Add water and set aside for 20 minutes or until tender. Drain. Transfer to a bowl. Stir in the lemon rind, lemon juice, chickpeas, mint and chives.

Spray a frying pan with olive oil spray. Add salmon and cook over medium-low heat for 4-5 minutes each side. Divide salad among serving plates and top with salmon. Serve with lemon wedges.

## Orange Fish

Serving 4
**List of Ingredients**
26.50 oz (750g) chat potatoes, halved

Olive oil cooking spray

3 slices white bread

1/4 cup fresh parsley, finely chopped

1 orange, rind finely grated

1 red chili, deseeded, finely chopped

4 thick, boneless white fish fillets

1 bunch asparagus, trimmed

Green salad, to serve

**Preparation**
Preheat oven to 392.00ºF (200°C). Line a baking tray with baking paper. Place potatoes, cut-side up, onto tray. Spray with oil. Season with salt. Bake for 25 minutes.

Process bread in a food processor to fine crumbs. Transfer to a bowl. Stir in parsley, rind and chili. Season with salt and pepper.

Spray fish with oil. Press crumb mixture onto fish. Spray with oil again. Place into oven below potatoes. Cook for 10 to 15 minutes or until fish is cooked through.

Cook asparagus in boiling water for 2 minutes or until bright green and tender. Drain. Serve with fish, potatoes and salad.

## Tabouli Fish

Serving 4
**List of Ingredients**
1 cup (170g) burghul

2 large vine ripened tomatoes, quartered, deseeded, finely chopped

1 Lebanese cucumber, halved lengthways, deseeded, finely chopped

1/4 cup chopped fresh continental parsley

1/4 cup chopped fresh mint

6 shallots, ends trimmed, pale section only, finely chopped

2 tbs fresh lemon juice

2 tsp olive oil

1/2 tsp ground cinnamon

Olive oil, extra, to grease

4 (about 5.30 oz or 150g each) firm white fish fillets (such as ling)

2 lemons, halved

**Preparation**

Place the burghul in a heatproof bowl. Add enough boiling water to cover. Set aside for 20 minutes to soak. Drain and remove as much liquid as possible. Transfer to a large bowl.

Stir in the tomato, cucumber, parsley, mint, shallot, lemon juice, oil and cinnamon. Taste and season with pepper.

Preheat a barbecue flat plate or large frying pan on high. Brush with oil to lightly grease. Add the fish and cook for 2 minutes each side or until the fish flakes easily when tested with a fork in the thickest part. Add the lemons, cut-side down, and cook for 1-2 minutes or until golden and caramelized.

Divide the tabouli among serving plates. Top with the fish and serve with the caramelized lemon.

## Mustard Trout and Caper

Serving 8
**List of Ingredients**
2 leeks, pale section only, washed, dried, quartered lengthways

2 lemons, thinly sliced

1 x 1kg side ocean trout, skin removed

1/5 cup (125ml) dry white wine

2 tbs water

1/5 cup (125ml) vegetable stock

4 green shallots, ends trimmed, thinly sliced

1 tbs Dijon mustard

2 tbs capers, rinsed, drained, coarsely chopped

Freshly ground black pepper

Green beans with almond & lemon dressing, to serve

Lemon slices, to serve

**Preparation**

Preheat oven to 338.00ºF (170°C). Place leek over the base of a large baking dish. Arrange half the lemon slices over the leek. Place trout on top of the leek mixture. Arrange remaining lemon slices over the trout.

Drizzle trout with 60ml (1/4 cup) of the wine and the water. Cover with foil and cook in preheated oven for 35 minutes or until cooked through. Remove from oven. Discard leek and lemon.

Meanwhile, combine the remaining wine, stock and shallot in a large frying pan over medium heat. Cook, stirring occasionally, for 3 minutes or until mixture is reduced by half. Remove from heat. Strain and discard the shallot. Return the wine mixture to the frying pan. Whisk in the mustard and capers. Taste and season with pepper.

Cut the trout into 8 equal portions. Divide the green beans with almond & lemon dressing among serving plates. Top with trout, lemon slices and mustard & caper dressing. Serve immediately.

# Red-Wine Salmon Lentils and Beetroot

Serving 6
**List of Ingredients**
2 tbs olive oil, plus extra to brush

1 onion, finely chopped

1 1/2 cups (300g) small whole green lentils, rinsed (see Notes)

2 tbs tomato paste

1L (4 cups) hot chicken or vegetable stock

2 cooked beetroot, peeled

2 tbs finely chopped flat-leaf parsley

28.20 oz (800g) piece salmon fillet, pin-boned

3 fresh or dried bay leaves

3.50 oz (100g) mache or watercress sprigs

**Red wine reduction**
750ml dry red wine

1 onion, finely chopped

2 garlic cloves, smashed

2 fresh or dried bay leaves

6 black peppercorns

## Preparation

For the reduction, place the list of ingredients in a wide saucepan and bring to the boil. Turn heat to medium-high and cook for 25 minutes or until reduced to 300ml. Strain, discard the solids and set aside.

Meanwhile, heat the olive oil in a large deep frypan over medium heat. Add the onion and cook for 10 minutes, stirring occasionally, until softened.

Add the lentils, tomato paste, stock and red wine reduction, and simmer over medium heat for 45 minutes or until the lentils are tender and the mixture is thick.

Finely chop the beetroot, reserving any juices, and add to the lentils with the parsley. Season to taste with sea salt and freshly ground black pepper, then heat through for a further 3 minutes.

Meanwhile, preheat the oven to 200C and line a roasting tray with foil.

Brush the salmon skin with the extra olive oil, arrange the bay leaves on top and place the salmon, skin-side, up on the roasting tray. Place in the oven and bake for 10 minutes (the salmon will still be a little opaque) or until it is cooked to your liking. Remove from the oven and allow to rest for 20 minutes.

Ladle the lentils onto 4 warmed plates. Cut the salmon into 4 pieces, discard the skin and bay leaves. Break the salmon into large bite-sized chunks and arrange on top of the lentils. Scatter with the lamb's lettuce or watercress to serve.

# Salmon Bean Mash

Serving 4
**List of Ingredients**
1 tbs olive oil

2 garlic cloves, crushed

1 tsp ground cumin

1 tsp finely grated lemon rind

2 x 14.10 oz (400g) cans cannellini beans, rinsed, drained

1 tbs fresh lemon juice

1 cup fresh continental parsley leaves

1 small red onion, halved, thinly sliced

1 tbs salted baby capers, rinsed, drained

Olive oil spray

4 (about 4.40 oz or 125g each) skinless salmon fillets

Steamed green round beans, to serve

**Preparation**
Heat the oil in a medium saucepan over medium heat. Add the garlic, cumin and lemon rind and cook, stirring, for 30 seconds or

until aromatic. Add the cannellini beans and lemon juice, and cook for 2 minutes. Use a fork to coarsely crush. Set aside and cover to keep warm.

Combine the parsley, onion and capers in a small bowl.

Heat a large non-stick frying pan over medium-high heat. Spray with oil. Cook the salmon for 3-4 minutes each side for medium or until cooked to your liking.

Divide the bean mixture among serving plates. Top with the salmon and the parsley mixture. Serve with green beans.

## Tuna Tabouli

Serving 4
**List of Ingredients**
1 1/2 cups (240g) burghul (cracked wheat)

2 x 15oz (425g) cans tuna in springwater, drained

8.80 oz (250g) punnet cherry tomatoes, halved

1 Lebanese cucumber, chopped into 1cm cubes

1 small red onion, thinly sliced

1/4 cup chopped flat-leaf parsley leaves

1/4 cup chopped dill

2 tbs extra virgin olive oil

2 tbs red wine vinegar

1 garlic clove, crushed

**Preparation**
Place the burghul in a bowl with 3 cups (750ml) cold water. Soak for 20 minutes or until softened. Drain well, squeezing out as much of the water as possible. Transfer the burghul to a large

bowl, then stir in the tuna, tomato, cucumber, red onion, parsley and dill.

Whisk the olive oil, vinegar and garlic together in a jug, then pour over the salad. Toss well to combine, then serve.

# Lime-Lemon Salmon

Serving 8

**List of Ingredients**

1.5kg whole side of salmon (1 large fillet)

1 lemon, thinly sliced

2 kaffir lime leaves, torn

1 lemongrass stalk, quartered, bruised

1 cup loosely packed fresh coriander leaves

Fresh coriander leaves, to serve

**Preparation**

Preheat oven to 356.00ºF/320.00ºF (180°C/160°C) fan-forced. Place foil sheets, slightly overlapping, on a large baking dish. Place salmon on foil. Top with lemon, lime leaves, lemongrass and coriander. Season with salt and pepper.

Bring 2 long sides of foil up to centre. Fold to seal. Roll up ends to enclose salmon. Bake for 30 minutes for medium or until cooked to your liking. Cool to room temperature. Cover. Refrigerate. Transfer to a platter. Top with coriander just before serving.

## Spicy Fish Kebabs with Fluffy Couscous

**List of Ingredients**
1/2 cup diced fresh coriander
1 lb fish fillets (firm, white, and skinless) – cut into 3cm pieces
1 cup chicken stock (reduced salt)
2 cloves garlic, crushed
1 tbsp olive oil
2 small red thai chilies, chopped
1/4 cup lemon juice
1/2 cup water
1 1/2 cups couscous
1/2 cup fresh coriander
1 tbsp preserved lemon, finely chopped
1/4 cup slivered almonds, toasted

**Preparation**
Place the oil, garlic, coriander, chili and lemon juice in a large bowl. Add fish pieces and coat with spice mix.
Using 8 skewers make kebabs out of the fish fillets (should make about 8) and place on a try. Cover and place in fridge for 40 minutes.
Heat an oiled grill plate (or barbeque) and allow kebabs to cook for about 5 minutes.
Pour stock and the water into a pot and bring to the boil. Remove from heat and add couscous. Cover and allow to stand for 5 minutes, or until the liquid is absorbed. After 5 minutes, fluff the couscous using a fork. Finish off by adding what was left of the coriander spice mix, coriander leaves, lemon and nuts to the couscous. Serve couscous with grilled fish kebabs

# Vegetable Salmon Salad

Serving 4
**List of Ingredients**
5.30 oz (150g) skinless salmon fillet

Olive oil spray

2 bunches asparagus, woody ends trimmed

1 large zucchini, trimmed, peeled into ribbons

14.10 oz (400g) can chickpeas, rinsed, and drained

1/2 small red onion, thinly sliced

1/2 cup fresh continental parsley leaves

5.30 oz (150g) couscous

150ml boiling water

1/3 cup (90g) low-fat natural yoghurt

1 tbs fresh lemon juice

2 tbs chopped fresh chives

**Preparation**

Preheat oven to 356.00ºF (180°C). Line a baking tray with non-stick baking paper. Bake salmon on tray for 8-10 minutes or until cooked through. Set aside to cool slightly. Flake into pieces.

Preheat a chargrill on high. Spray lightly with oil. Cook the asparagus and zucchini for 2 minutes each side or until charred and tender crisp. Transfer to a plate. Halve the asparagus lengthways. Combine salmon, asparagus, zucchini, chickpeas, onion and parsley in a bowl.

Place couscous in a heatproof bowl. Add water. Cover with plastic wrap. Set aside for 3-4 minutes or until liquid is absorbed. Use a fork to separate grains.

Whisk yoghurt, lemon juice and chives in a bowl. Divide couscous and salmon mixture among plates. Drizzle over dressing.

# Beef and Veal Recipes

## Balsamic Green Beans and Beef

Serving 8

**List of Ingredients**

2.2 lbs (1kg) orange sweet potato (kumara), peeled, cut into 2cm pieces

1 tsp olive oil

4 (about 4.40 oz or 125g each) beef fillet steaks, excess fat trimmed

1/2 cup (125ml) balsamic vinegar

1/4 cup (60ml) salt-reduced beef stock

1/4 cup (60ml) water

8 fresh corn cobbettes

8.80 oz (250g) green beans, topped

**Preparation**

Place the sweet potato in a large saucepan and cover with cold water. Bring to the boil over high heat and cook for 10 minutes or until tender. Drain and use a potato masher or fork to mash until smooth. Season with pepper.

Meanwhile, heat the oil in a large non-stick frying pan over medium-high heat. Add the steaks and cook for 2-3 minutes each side for medium or until cooked to your liking. Transfer to a plate and cover loosely with foil. Set aside for 5 minutes to rest. Add the vinegar, stock and water to the pan. Bring to the boil over high heat. Boil, uncovered, for 6-7 minutes or until the mixture reduces and thickens slightly.

While the sauce is cooking, place the corn in a steamer basket over saucepan of simmering water. Steam, covered, for 5 minutes. Add the green beans to the basket with the corn and steam, covered, for a further 4 minutes or until the vegetables are just tender.

Divide the sweet potato mash among serving plates. Top with the steak and drizzle over the balsamic sauce. Serve with the steamed corn and green beans.

# Lentil Beef Burger

Serving 4
**List of Ingredients**
14.10 oz (400g) can Annalisa Lentils, rinsed, and drained

10.60 oz (300g) lean beef mince

1 small zucchini, coarsely grated

1 egg

8.80 oz (250g) cherry tomatoes, halved

2 tbs chopped fresh coriander

Olive oil spray

1/3 cup (90g) low-fat hummus

4 wholegrain rolls, split, toasted

1 Lebanese cucumber, trimmed, thinly sliced

2 cups (80g) baby spinach leaves

**Preparation**
Place the lentils, mince, zucchini and egg in a large bowl. Season with salt and pepper. Use clean hands to mix until well combined.

Shape into 4 patties. Place on a baking tray. Cover and place in the fridge for 10 minutes to chill.

Meanwhile, combine the tomato and coriander in a bowl.

Spray a barbecue grill or chargrill with oil and heat on medium-high. Cook the patties for 4 minutes each side or until lightly charred and cooked through. Spread the hummus over the base of each roll. Top with the cucumber, spinach, patties, tomato mixture and remaining roll.

# Beef Kebabs Couscous and Chickpea

Serving 4
**List of Ingredients**
1 lemon

1 cup (190g) couscous

1 cup (250ml) boiling water

2 tsp olive oil

14.10 oz (400g) beef rump steak, excess fat trimmed, cut into long thin strips

2 tsp ground cumin

1 x 14.10 oz (400g) can chickpeas, rinsed, drained

2 tomatoes, coarsely chopped

2 shallots, ends trimmed, thinly sliced

1/2 cup fresh mint leaves, coarsely chopped

1/2 cup fresh continental parsley leaves, coarsely chopped

**Preparation**
Use a zester to remove the rind from the lemon. (Alternatively, use a vegetable peeler to peel the rind from the lemon. Use a

small sharp knife to remove the white pith from the rind. Cut the rind into very thin strips.) Juice the lemon.

Place the couscous in a large heatproof bowl. Combine the water and oil, and add to the couscous. Cover and set aside for 5 minutes or until all the liquid is absorbed. Use a fork to separate the grains.

Meanwhile, thread the beef onto 8 skewers. Sprinkle the kebabs with the cumin.

Add the lemon zest, lemon juice, chickpeas, tomato, shallot, mint and parsley to the couscous. Toss until well combined.

Heat a barbecue grill over medium-high heat. Add the skewers and cook for 3 minutes each side for medium or until cooked to your liking. Divide the skewers and couscous tabouli among serving plates and serve.

# Ginger Beef Stir-Fry

Serving 4

**List of Ingredients**

12.40 oz (350g) lean beef sirloin steak, sliced on the diagonal

1 teaspoon sesame oil

6cm piece ginger, thinly sliced

Olive oil cooking spray

4 green onions, sliced on the diagonal

7.10 oz (200g) snow peas, trimmed, sliced in half on the diagonal

5.30 oz (150g) oyster mushrooms, chopped

1 red capsicum, sliced

4.20 oz (120g) baby corn, sliced in half on the diagonal

2 tablespoons reduced-salt soy sauce

Cooked brown rice, to serve

**Preparation**

Place steak, sesame oil and ginger into a shallow ceramic dish.

Cover and refrigerate for 30 minutes if time permits.

Heat a wok over high heat until hot. Spray with oil. Add one-third of the beef. Stir-fry for 1 minute or until browned. Remove to a plate. Repeat twice with remaining beef, spraying wok each time.

Spray wok lightly with oil. Add vegetables and stir-fry for 3 minutes or until just tender.

Return beef to the wok with soy sauce. Stir-fry for 1 minute or until heated through. Serve with brown rice.

# Rocket Beef Wrap

Serving 4

**List of Ingredients**

1 x 14.10 oz (400g) can chickpeas, rinsed, drained

1 tbs tahini (sesame paste)

1 garlic clove, chopped

2 tbs fresh lemon juice

1/2 tsp ground cumin

4 pieces whole meal lavash

8.80 oz (250g) sliced rare roast beef

1 cup (200g) 97 per cent fat-free semi-dried tomatoes, chopped

1 bunch rocket, stems trimmed, washed, and dried

**Preparation**

Place chickpeas, tahini, garlic, lemon juice and cumin in the bowl of a food processor and process until smooth.

Place the lavash on a clean work surface. Spread evenly with chickpea mixture, and top with roast beef, semi-dried tomato and rocket.

Roll up lavash to enclose filling. Cut in half diagonally and serve immediately.

## Veal Salad

Serving 4

**List of Ingredients**

1/2 cup fresh continental parsley leaves

1/2 cup fresh basil leaves, torn

2 tbs fresh mint leaves

1 tbs baby capers, rinsed

1 tbs red wine vinegar

2 tsp olive oil

Olive oil spray

4 (about 4.40 oz or 125g each) veal steaks

2 x 14.10 oz (400g) cans Butter Beans, rinsed, drained

1 x 8.80 oz (250g) punnet grape tomatoes, halved

2 garlic cloves, crushed

**Preparation**

Combine the parsley, basil, mint, capers, vinegar and oil in a small bowl.

Spray a large frying pan with olive oil spray to grease. Heat over medium-high heat.

Season both sides of the veal with salt and pepper. Cook for 2 minutes each side for medium or until cooked to your liking. Transfer to a plate and cover with foil. Set aside for 5 minutes to rest.

Add the beans, tomato and garlic to the pan and cook, stirring, for 2 minutes or until the beans are heated through. Stir in half the parsley mixture.

Divide the bean mixture among serving dishes. Top with the veal. Top with remaining parsley mixture to serve.

## Veal Garlic Chickpeas

Serving 4

**List of Ingredients**

2 x 14.10 oz (400g) cans chickpeas, drained, rinsed

5.30 oz (150g) cherry tomatoes, quartered

2 green onions, thinly sliced

1 garlic clove, crushed

2 tablespoons lemon juice

olive oil cooking spray

4 (4.40 oz or 125g each) veal loin chops

**Gremolata**

1/3 cup chopped fresh flat-leaf parsley leaves

2 teaspoons finely grated lemon rind

**Preparation**

Make gremolata: Combine parsley and lemon rind in a bowl. Set aside.

Place chickpeas in a large bowl. Add tomatoes, onions, garlic and lemon juice. Toss to combine.

Spray a frying pan with oil. Heat over medium-high heat. Cook veal for 5 to 6 minutes each side or until browned and cooked to your liking. Serve veal with chickpea mixture and gremolata.

# Lamb Recipes

## Spiced Tabouli Lamb

**List of Ingredients**

1 cup (160g) burghul (cracked wheat) (see note)

2 tsp ground cumin

Olive oil spray

2 x 8.80 oz (250g) lamb backstraps, trimmed

2 tomatoes, seeds removed, chopped

1 Lebanese cucumber, chopped

4 spring onions, finely chopped

1 cup chopped flat-leaf parsley

1 tbs extra virgin olive oil

Juice of 1/2 lemon

1 garlic clove, crushed

1/3 cup (95g) low-fat tzatziki

**Preparation**

Toast burghul in a large, dry fry pan over medium heat for 2-3 minutes, stirring occasionally. Transfer to a bowl and cover with boiling water by about 5cm. Soak for 10 minutes, then drain excess water.

Meanwhile, combine cumin with a little salt and pepper on a plate. Spray lamb with oil and coat in cumin mixture.

Heat a pan over medium-high heat and cook lamb for 3-4 minutes each side until browned but still pink in the centre (or until done to your liking). Wrap loosely in foil and rest while you finish the tabouli.

Stir the tomato, cucumber, onion and parsley into the burghul. Whisk together oil, lemon juice and garlic, stir through burghul, and then season to taste.

Thinly slice the lamb and serve with the tabouli and tzatziki.

# Almond Lamb Pilaf

Serving 4
**List of Ingredients**
1 1/2 tbs olive oil

1 brown onion, finely chopped

2 garlic cloves, crushed

1 tbs boiling water

Pinch of saffron threads

2 1/2 cups (625ml) salt-reduced chicken stock

1 x 7cm cinnamon stick

1 1/2 cups (300g) basmati rice

1/4 cup (25g) flaked almonds

7.10 oz (200g) cup mushrooms, thinly sliced

14.10 oz (400g) lamb eye of loin (backstrap)

1 bunch asparagus, woody ends trimmed, cut into 2cm pieces

1 cup (150g) frozen peas

2 ripe tomatoes, coarsely chopped

1/4 cup chopped fresh continental parsley

## Preparation

Heat 1 tablespoon of oil in a large saucepan over medium heat. Add the onion and garlic and cook, stirring occasionally, for 4 minutes or until the onion softens.

Meanwhile, combine the water and saffron in a small bowl. Place the stock and cinnamon in a medium saucepan over medium heat. Bring to a simmer.

Add rice to the onion mixture. Cook, stirring, for 2 minutes. Add the saffron mixture and the stock mixture. Bring to a simmer. Reduce heat to low. Cover and cook, without stirring, for 12 minutes.

While the rice is cooking, place the almonds in a large frying pan over medium heat and cook, stirring, for 3 minutes or until toasted. Transfer to a large plate. Heat the remaining oil in the frying pan over medium-high heat. Add the mushroom and cook for 4 minutes or until tender. Transfer to the plate with the almonds. Add the lamb to the pan and cook for 3 minutes each side for medium or until cooked to your liking. Transfer to the plate.

Add asparagus, peas and tomato to the rice. Set aside, covered, for 5 minutes.

Thickly slice the lamb across the grain. Add the lamb, almonds, mushroom and parsley to the rice mixture and combine. Season with salt and pepper to serve.

## Lentil Lamb Salad

Serving 4
**List of Ingredients**
1 x 7.10 oz (200g) punnet grape tomatoes

2 tsp olive oil

1 brown onion, halved, finely chopped

2 garlic cloves, crushed

1/4 tsp cayenne pepper

5.30 oz (150g) cup mushrooms, thickly sliced

1 x 14.10 oz (400g) can brown lentils, rinsed, and drained

1 tbs balsamic vinegar

1.40 oz (40g) baby spinach leaves

12 (about 34.40 oz or 975g) lamb cutlets, excess fat trimmed

**Preparation**
Cut a small slit in each tomato. Heat half the oil in a large non-stick frying pan over medium heat. Add the onion and cook, stirring occasionally, for 5 minutes or until soft. Add the garlic and

cayenne pepper and cook, stirring, for 30 seconds or until aromatic.

Add the mushroom and tomatoes and cook, stirring occasionally, for 5 minutes or until mushroom and tomatoes soften. Add the lentils and vinegar and cook, tossing gently, for 2 minutes or until heated through. Transfer to a large heatproof bowl. Add the spinach and gently stir until just combined.

Wipe the pan clean with paper towel. Heat the remaining oil in the pan over medium-high heat. Add the lamb and cook for 3 minutes each side for medium or until cooked to your liking. Transfer to a plate and cover with foil. Set aside for 5 minutes to rest.

Divide the lentil salad among serving plates and top with the lamb cutlets. Serve immediately.

## Lemon Lamb and Vegetables

Serving 4
**List of Ingredients**
1 tbs extra virgin olive oil

1 lemon, rind finely grated, juiced

1 tbs coarsely chopped fresh rosemary

1 tbs coarsely chopped fresh oregano

1 large garlic clove, crushed

1 tsp water

Salt & freshly ground black pepper

4 x 4.40 oz (125g) lamb leg steaks, excess fat trimmed

10.60 oz (300g) broad beans, shelled

1 bunch asparagus, woody ends trimmed, cut in half diagonally

7.10 oz (200g) green beans, topped, halved crossways

14.10 oz (400g) fresh peas, shelled

2 tbs chicken stock or water

1 small fresh red chili, deseeded, finely chopped

1 tbs capers, rinsed, drained, finely chopped

## Preparation

Combine 2 tsp of the oil with the lemon juice, rosemary, oregano, garlic and water in a large glass or ceramic bowl. Season with pepper. Add the lamb and turn to evenly coat. Cover with plastic wrap and place in the fridge for 30 minutes to develop the flavors.

Cook the broad beans in a small saucepan of salted boiling water for 5 minutes or until tender. Drain. Refresh under cold running water. Remove skins and set aside in a bowl.

Preheat a chargrill on high. Heat the remaining oil in a medium frying pan over medium-high heat. Add the asparagus, beans and peas, and cook, tossing gently, for 4 minutes or until bright green and tender crisp. Add the broad beans, stock or water, lemon rind, chili and capers, and season with salt and pepper. Gently toss for a further 1 minute. Remove from heat. Transfer to a bowl and cover with foil to keep warm.

Cook lamb steaks on preheated grill for 3 minutes each side for medium-rare or until cooked to your liking.

Spoon the bean mixture among serving plates. Top with lamb and serve immediately.

# Lamb Barley Salad

**List of Ingredients**

1 tbsp crushed coriander seeds

1/2 tsp dried chili flakes

2 cloves crushed garlic

1 lb lamb back straps

1 cup pearl barley

1/4 teaspoon ground turmeric

1/3 cup each loosely packed fresh mint and coriander leaves

1 chopped small red onion

1 cup cherry tomatoes – cut in half

1/4 cup lemon juice

2 tsp olive oil

**Preparation**

Make the lamb spice by combining the chili, garlic and seeds. Once combined rub spice all over lamb. Place in the refrigerator for 30 min.

Place barley in large pot and boil for approximately 20 min. Rinse and drain once cooked.

Cook lamb on a grill to your liking. Once done put to one side and allow to stand for few minutes before slicing into thick pieces.

Place the rest of the List of Ingredients in a large bowl and add cooked barley.

Serve tender pieces of lamb with barley salad.

# Pork Recipes

## Rosemary Pork and Pears

Serving 4
**List of Ingredients**
4 Beurre Bosc pears, unpeeled, cored, cut into 2cm-thick wedges

2 red onions, cut into thick wedges

Olive oil spray

2 tbs balsamic vinegar

2 tbs wholegrain mustard

2 tsp chopped fresh rosemary

1 tsp finely grated lemon rind

1 tbs olive oil

4 (about 4.40 oz or 125g each) pork loin steaks

100g baby spinach leaves

Steamed green round beans, to serve

## Preparation

Preheat oven to 392.00ºF (200°C). Line two baking trays with non-stick baking paper. Place pear and onion on one of the trays. Spray with oil. Drizzle with half the vinegar. Bake for 25 minutes or until the pears are golden and tender.

Meanwhile, combine the mustard, rosemary and lemon rind in a bowl. Heat the olive oil in a large non-stick frying pan over high heat. Cook the pork for 2 minutes each side or until golden. Remove from heat. Spread one side of each pork steak with mustard mixture. Transfer to the second baking tray. Bake for 6-7 minutes or until cooked through.

Place the pear, onion, spinach and remaining vinegar in a bowl, and toss to combine.

Divide pear mixture and pork steaks among serving plates. Serve with beans.

# Mustard Orange Pork

Serving 4
**List of Ingredients**
17.60 oz (500g) carrots, peeled, cut into 3cm pieces

17.60 oz (500g) orange sweet potato, peeled, cut into 3cm pieces

Olive oil cooking spray

4 (3.50 oz or 100g each) pork butterfly steaks, trimmed

3 oranges, juiced

3/4 cup salt-reduced chicken stock

1 tablespoon wholegrain mustard

1 teaspoon yellow box honey

7.10 oz (200g) green beans, steamed, to serve

**Preparation**
Place carrots and sweet potato in a saucepan and cover with cold water. Cover and bring to the boil over high heat. Reduce heat to medium. Cook, partially covered, for 12 to 15 minutes or until tender. Drain and return to saucepan. Mash until almost smooth. Season with pepper.

Meanwhile, spray a large, non-stick frying pan with oil. Heat over medium heat. Add pork and cook for 1 to 1 1/2 minutes (depending on thickness) each side or until just cooked through. Transfer to a plate. Cover loosely with foil and set aside for 5 minutes to rest.

Add 3/4 cup orange juice, stock, mustard and honey to pan. Stir to remove sediment from base of pan. Increase heat to high. Cook for 8 to 10 minutes or until sauce reduces and thickens. Season with pepper.

Spoon mash onto plates. Top with pork and spoon over sauce. Serve with beans.

## Pork Burritos

Serving 4
**List of Ingredients**
1 tbs olive oil

17.60 oz (500g) pork loin steaks, thinly sliced

1 red onion, halved, thinly sliced

2 tsp sweet paprika

2 tsp ground coriander

1 x 14.10 oz (400g) can chopped tomatoes

1 x 14.10 oz (400g) can red kidney beans, rinsed, drained

2 tbs chopped fresh coriander

8 flour tortillas

Shredded iceberg lettuce, to serve

Natural yoghurt, to serve

**Preparation**
Heat half the oil in a large non-stick frying pan over high heat. Add half the pork and cook, stirring, for 3 minutes or until golden.

Transfer to a plate. Repeat with the remaining pork, reheating the pan between batches.

Heat the remaining oil in the pan. Add the onion and cook, stirring, for 2 minutes or until light golden. Add the paprika and coriander and cook, stirring, for 1 minute. Add the tomato and beans. Bring to the boil. Reduce heat to medium-high. Simmer for 3 minutes.

Return the pork to the pan. Simmer for 1 minute or until heated through. Remove from heat. Stir in the coriander.

Spoon a little of the pork mixture along the centre of each tortilla. Top with the lettuce and a dollop of yoghurt. Roll up to enclose the filling. Serve.

## Pork Skewers

Serving 4
**List of Ingredients**
12 pre-soaked bamboo skewers.

17.60 oz (500g) extra-trim pork loin steaks, cut into 2cm cubes

1 tablespoon Middle Eastern seasoning

17.60 oz (500g) eggplant, cut into 2cm cubes

1 large red capsicum, cut into 2cm cubes

10.60 oz (300g) zucchini, cut into 2cm cubes

17.60 oz (500g) jap pumpkin, peeled, cut into 2cm cubes

Olive oil cooking spray

1/2 cup burghul (cracked wheat)

1 cup boiling water

2 tablespoons chopped fresh flat-leaf parsley leaves

2 tablespoons chopped fresh coriander leaves

1 1/2 tablespoons fat-free Italian dressing

Lemon wedges, to serve

**Preparation**

Preheat oven to 428.00ºF/392.00ºF (220°C/200°C) fan-forced. Line 2 roasting trays with baking paper.

Place pork and seasoning in a shallow glass or ceramic dish. Stir to coat. Thread pork onto skewers. Cover and refrigerate.

Divide eggplant, capsicum, zucchini and pumpkin between prepared trays. Spray with oil. Roast for 30 to 40 minutes or until tender and light golden.

Meanwhile, place burghul in a large, heatproof bowl. Cover with boiling water. Set aside for 10 minutes. Drain. Using hands, squeeze out excess liquid. Return to bowl.

Spray a barbecue plate or chargrill with oil. Heat over medium heat. Cook skewers for 2 minutes each side or until cooked through.

Add roasted vegetables, parsley, coriander and dressing to burghul. Season with salt and pepper. Toss to combine. Serve skewers with burghul mixture and lemon wedges.

## Asian Pork

Serving 6
**List of Ingredients**
Olive oil spray

17.60 oz (500g) lean pork loin medallion steaks

1 large carrot, peeled, cut into thin matchsticks

1 small red onion, halved, thinly sliced

3.50 oz (100g) bean sprouts, trimmed

3.50 oz (100g) snow peas, thinly sliced lengthways

1/2 small wombok (Chinese cabbage), finely shredded

1 cup chopped fresh coriander

1 tbs finely shredded fresh ginger

3 tsp sesame oil

3 tsp salt-reduced soy sauce

2 tsp honey

1 garlic clove, crushed

**Preparation**

Heat a large frying pan over medium-high heat. Spray with oil. Cook the pork for 2-3 minutes each side or until golden and just cooked through. Transfer to a plate. Cover with foil and set aside for 5 minutes to rest. Thinly slice across the grain.

Meanwhile, combine the carrot, onion, bean sprouts, snow peas, wombok, coriander and ginger in a large bowl.

To make the dressing, whisk the oil, soy sauce, honey and garlic in a small jug.

Add the pork to the salad. Drizzle over the dressing and toss to combine.

## Pork Tenderloin

**List of Ingredients**
2 pork tenderloins
2 tbsp chili powder
¼ tsp of ground ginger, thyme and pepper (1/4 tsp of each)
1 tsp salt

**Preparation**
In a small bowl combine all the spices.
Run the spices all over the tenderloin to season. Cover and place in the fridge for a few hours.
Grill tenderloins over medium heat for 30 to 40 minutes until cooked through.

## Orange Pork Chops

**List of Ingredients**
6 thick pork loin chops
1 tbsp vegetable oil
1 Tbsp Stevia powdered extract (1 tsp Stevia liquid concentrate)
¾ cup water
½ tsp pepper
½ tsp paprika
1 ¼ tsp salt
1 orange (zest and then peel and cut into pieces)
1 cup orange juice (fresh)
1 tbsp cornstarch
12 cloves
½ tsp cinnamon

**Preparation**
In a large pan heat oil and then brown pork on both sides. Now add the water, salt, paprika, and pepper and bring to a boil. Turn down the heat and allow to cook for 40 minutes. Turn the chops at least once during this time.

In a separate saucepan add orange juice, 1 tbsp orange zest, Stevia starch, cloves, cinnamon and leftover salt. Allow to cook until thick and then add orange pieces.

Pour this delicious sauce over your pork chops and serve with vegetables of your choice

## Berry Pork Roast

**List of Ingredients**
1 large pork loin
2 cups raspberries
2 cups blackberries
1 tsp thyme
2 tbsp of crushed pecans

**Preparation**
Place blackberries and raspberries in a blender and blend until liquid consistency has formed.
Preheat your oven to 392 deg. F (200 deg. Celsius).
Place pork in oven pan and Rub thyme all over before topping with liquidized berries.
Cover foil and bake for approximately 4 hours or until loin is tender.
Serve with your favourite vegetables.

# Pork and Veggies Cabbage Rolls

**List of Ingredients**
7 oz. lean minced pork
2 cups cooked brown rice
8 big cabbage leaves
1 tsp olive oil
1 large carrot, grated
1 chopped brown onion
1 finely diced celery stalk
1 tbsp tomato paste
2 tsp ground cumin
1 tsp ground coriander
1/2 tsp ground allspice
2 crushed garlic cloves
1/3 cup baby rocket leaves
**Tomato Sauce**
1 1/2 cups canned crushed tomatoes
1/2 cup chicken stock (reduced salt)
2 crushed cloves garlic
1 tbsp shredded fresh flat-leaf parsley
**Preparation**

Cook cabbage leaves by either steaming or boiling. Once cooked, rinse and drain and place on absorbent paper to get rid of excess moisture.

In a large saucepan fry onions, carrots, celery and garlic for about 5 min. Now add paste and pork and keep frying until pork has browned.

Once the pork has browned add the remaining spices and stir to combine.

Slowly stir in rice. Now remove from heat and allow to cool for a few minutes.

Distribute the rice mixture amongst the cabbage leaves and carefully roll each one making sure to fold in all edges.
Cook the rolls for 10 minutes over either a bamboo steamer lined with baking paper or over a large pot of simmering water. Each roll must be cooked and heated all the way through.
To make tomato sauce, place undrained tomatoes, garlic and stock in a small pan. Once the mixture starts to boil, reduce heat and simmer uncovered for about 10 minutes. Once done stir in parsley
.

# Salad Recipes

## Nut Bean Salad

Serving 4

**List of Ingredients**

2 tablespoons pine nuts

4.40 oz (125g) green beans, trimmed

1 bunch asparagus, trimmed

1/4 cup French dressing

**Preparation**

Preheat oven to 356°F/320°F (180°C/160°C) fan-forced. Place pine nuts on a baking tray. Bake for 4 to 5 minutes or until golden.

Cook beans and asparagus in a saucepan of boiling water for 2 minutes or until just tender. Drain. Refresh under cold water.

Place pine nuts, beans and asparagus in a large bowl. Add dressing. Toss to combine. Serve.

# Vegetable Bean Salad

Serving 6
**List of Ingredients**
1 medium red capsicum, thickly sliced

1 medium yellow capsicum, thickly sliced

2 medium zucchini, cut diagonally into 1cm-thick slices

3.50 oz (100g) button mushrooms, halved

1 medium red onion, cut into wedges

1 tablespoon olive oil

2 tablespoons balsamic vinegar

2 garlic cloves, crushed

8.80 oz (250g) cherry tomatoes

7.10 oz (200g) green beans, trimmed

2 tablespoons pine nuts, toasted

**Preparation**
Preheat oven to 392.00ºF/356.00ºF (200°C/180°C). Place capsicum, zucchini, mushrooms and onion in a large baking dish.

Combine oil, vinegar and garlic in a bowl. Drizzle over vegetables. Toss to coat.

Roast for 20 minutes. Add tomatoes. Roast for 15 minutes or until vegetables are tender and tomatoes are starting to collapse.

Meanwhile, bring a large saucepan of water to the boil over high heat. Cook beans for 3 minutes or until bright green and just tender. Drain. Refresh in a bowl of iced water. Drain. Pat dry with paper towel.

Add beans to vegetable mixture. Toss to combine. Sprinkle with pine nuts. Season with salt and pepper. Serve.

## Bean Salad and Vegies

Serving 4
**List of Ingredients**
1 10.60 oz (300g) eggplant, halved lengthways
2 corn cobs, trimmed, cut into 2cm rounds
2 medium zucchini, thickly sliced diagonally
1 red capsicum, thickly sliced
1/3 cup olive oil
1 1/2 tablespoons chopped fresh oregano leaves
2 x 14.10 oz (400g) cans borlotti beans, drained, rinsed
2.10 oz (60g) baby rocket
1 tablespoon white balsamic vinegar
**Preparation**
Place cut-side of eggplant on board. Cut each half into 5mm-thick slices. Heat a greased barbecue plate or chargrill over medium heat. Combine eggplant, corn, zucchini, capsicum, oil and oregano in a bowl. Season with salt and pepper.

Chargrill vegetables, in batches, for 2 to 3 minutes each side or until tender. Transfer to a bowl. Add beans, rocket and vinegar. Toss to combine. Serve.

# Nutty Broccoli Lentil Salad

Serving 4

**List of Ingredients**

21.20 oz (600g) broccoli, trimmed, cut into florets

1 x 14.10 oz (400g) can brown lentils, rinsed, and drained

2 tsp balsamic vinegar

1 tbs olive oil

6 shallots, ends trimmed, thinly sliced

1 long fresh red chili, deseeded, finely chopped

2 garlic cloves, thinly sliced

2.60 oz (75g) baby spinach leaves

2 tbs toasted pine nuts

**Preparation**

Cook the broccoli in a large saucepan of boiling water for 3-4 minutes or until bright green and tender crisp. Refresh under cold running water. Drain.

Place the lentils in a bowl. Whisk together the vinegar and 2 teaspoons of olive oil. Add to lentils. Stir to combine.

Heat the remaining oil in a large non-stick frying pan over medium heat. Add the shallot, chili and garlic. Cook, stirring, for 1 minute or until aromatic. Add the broccoli and cook, stirring occasionally, for 2 minutes or until heated through and the broccoli is coated in the shallot mixture.

Add the broccoli mixture and spinach to the lentil mixture. Season with pepper. Toss to combine.

Divide the salad among serving bowls. Sprinkle with the pine nuts to serve.

# Barley Rice Salad

Serving 4

**List of Ingredients**

2/3 cup (140g) brown rice

2/3 cup (150g) pearl barley

1 red onion, cut into thick wedges

3 zucchini, trimmed, thickly sliced

1 red capsicum, deseeded, cut into 1.5cm pieces

Olive oil spray

2.60 oz (75g) baby spinach leaves

2 tbs currants

1/4 cup chopped fresh coriander

**Tahini Dressing**

1/4 cup (60ml) low fat natural yoghurt

2 tbs fresh lemon juice

1 tbs hot water

2 tsp tahini

1 tsp honey

**Preparation**
Preheat oven to 356.00ºF (180°C). Line a large baking tray with non-stick baking paper.

Cook the brown rice and pearl barley in a large saucepan of boiling water for 25 minutes or until tender. Drain.

Meanwhile: place the onion, zucchini and capsicum in a single layer on the lined tray and lightly spray with oil spray. Bake in oven for 25-30 minutes or until vegetables are tender.

Place the rice, barley, onion mixture, baby spinach, currants and coriander in a large bowl and gently toss until just combined. Season with pepper.

To make the tahini dressing: whisk together the yoghurt, lemon juice, water, tahini and honey in a medium bowl.

Spoon the salad among serving plates. Drizzle with tahini dressing to serve.

## Tofu Rice Salad

Serving 4

**List of Ingredients**

1 cup (200g) brown rice

2 celery sticks, trimmed, thinly sliced

1 small red capsicum, halved, deseeded, coarsely chopped

2.60 oz (75g) baby spinach leaves

2 tbs currants

1/4 cup (40g) sunflower seed kernels

7.10 oz (200g) Soyco Japanese Tofu (see note), thinly sliced

**Dressing**

2 tbs fresh orange juice

1 1/2 tbs salt-reduced soy sauce

2 tsp honey

2 tsp freshly grated ginger

**Preparation**

Cook the rice in a large saucepan of boiling water following packet directions. Rinse under cold running water. Drain.

To make the dressing, combine the orange juice, soy sauce, honey and ginger in a small bowl.

Place the rice, celery, capsicum, spinach, currants and half the sunflower seeds in a large bowl. Drizzle over the dressing and toss to combine.

Divide the rice mixture among serving bowls and top with the tofu. Sprinkle with the remaining sunflower seeds to serve.

# Pumpkin Rice Eggplant Salad

Serving 4

**List of Ingredients**

28.20 oz (800g) pumpkin, peeled, seeded, cut into 1.5cm pieces

1 medium (about 15.90 oz or 450g) eggplant, ends trimmed, cut into 1.5cm pieces

2 tsp ground cumin

Olive oil spray

3 cups (525g) cooked brown rice

1 zucchini, trimmed, halved, thinly sliced

1/4 cup (45g) pepitas, lightly toasted

1/4 cup fresh continental parsley leaves, chopped

1/4 cup fresh mint leaves, torn

1/4 cup (45g) currants

1/2 cup (130g) low-fat natural yoghurt

1 garlic clove, crushed

1 1/2 tbs fresh lemon juice

**Preparation**

Preheat oven to 200ºC. Line a baking tray with non-stick baking paper. Place pumpkin and eggplant on prepared tray. Sprinkle with cumin and season with pepper. Spray with oil and roast for 25 minutes or until tender.

Combine the pumpkin, eggplant, rice, zucchini, pepitas, parsley, mint and currants in a large bowl.

Combine the yoghurt, garlic and lemon juice in a small bowl. Divide salad among serving bowls and top with dressing.

# Rice Pumpkin and Seed Salad

Serving 4
**List of Ingredients**
Olive oil spray, to grease

2.2 lbs (1kg) kent pumpkin, peeled, deseeded, cut into 2-3cm pieces

2 cups (400g) long-grain brown rice

1/3 cup (60g) pepitas (pumpkin seed kernels)

1/3 cup (55g) sunflower seed kernels

1/3 cup (80ml) fresh lime juice

1 tbs soy sauce

1/2 tsp sesame oil

1 small garlic clove, crushed

1/4 tsp brown sugar

1 bunch rocket, washed, trimmed, leaves torn

**Preparation**
Preheat oven to 392.00ºF (200°C). Spray a large baking tray with olive oil to lightly grease. Arrange the pumpkin, in a single layer,

on the prepared tray and spray lightly with olive oil. Bake in preheated oven, turning halfway through cooking, for 30 minutes or until light brown and tender. Remove from oven and set aside for 15 minutes to cool to room temperature.

Meanwhile: cook the rice in a large saucepan of boiling water for 30 minutes or until tender (do not overcook). Drain in a large colander and set aside for 30 minutes to cool to room temperature.

Reduce oven temperature to 180°C. Spread the pepitas and sunflower seed kernels over a large baking tray. Bake in oven, stirring halfway through cooking, for 5 minutes or until lightly toasted. Remove from oven and set aside to cool slightly.

Combine the lime juice, soy sauce, sesame oil, garlic and sugar in a small jug. Place the rice in a large bowl. Drizzle with lime-juice mixture and use a large metal spoon to gently stir until well combined. Add the rocket, pumpkin, pepitas and sunflower seed kernels to the rice mixture and gently stir until well combined. Spoon salad among serving plates and serve immediately.

## Salad Cups

Serving 4

**List of Ingredients**

40g (1/4 cup) burghul (cracked wheat)

7.10 oz (200g) grape tomatoes, thinly sliced

2 salad onions, thinly sliced

2 tbs roughly chopped mint leaves

1/2 cup roughly chopped cherbil or flat leaf parsley

2 tbs lemon juice

2 tsp olive oil

14.10 oz (400g) can soy beans, rinsed, and drained

4 large butter lettuce leaves

**Preparation**

Place the burghul in a bowl, pour over 125ml (1/2 cup) boiling water, and soak for 10 minutes. Drain well, then use your hands to squeeze out any excess moisture.

Place the brughul, in a large bowl with the tomatoes, onion, mint, chervil or parsley, lemon juice, oil and beans. Season to taste with salt and pepper, then toss well.

Place a lettuce leaf on each plate, spoon the burghul mixture on top and serve.

## Lemon Bean Salad

Serving 8
**List of Ingredients**
2 x 14.10 oz (400g) cans cannellini beans, drained, rinsed

14.10 oz (400g) can chickpeas, drained, rinsed

14.10 oz (400g) can lentils, drained, rinsed

1/2 cup chopped fresh flat-leaf parsley leaves

1 tablespoon finely chopped fresh chives

**Dressing**
2 teaspoons finely grated lemon rind

1 tablespoon lemon juice

2 tablespoons olive oil

1 small garlic clove, crushed

**Preparation**
Combine beans, chickpeas, lentils, parsley and chives in a bowl.

Make dressing Place lemon rind, lemon juice, oil and garlic in a screw-top jar. Season with salt and pepper. Secure lid. Shake to combine. Toss dressing through salad. Serve.

## Parsley Bean Salad

Serving 4
**List of Ingredients**
1 x 14.10 oz (400g) can cannellini beans, rinsed, drained

1 x 8.80 oz (250g) punnet cherry tomatoes, halved

1 bunch fresh continental parsley, washed, leaves picked

1/2 small red onion, cut into thin wedges

2 tbs red wine vinegar

2 tsp extra virgin olive oil

1 garlic clove, crushed

Salt & freshly ground black pepper

**Preparation**
Place the cannellini beans, tomato, parsley and onion in a large bowl and toss to combine.

Whisk together the vinegar, oil and garlic in a small jug until well combined. Taste and season with salt and pepper. Drizzle the cannellini bean mixture with dressing and toss until well combined. Serve immediately.

## Bean Tomato Salad

Serving 5
**List of Ingredients**
14.10 oz (400g) can cannellini beans, drained, rinsed

1/2 small red onion, finely chopped

7.10 oz (200g) grape tomatoes, halved

2 tablespoons red wine vinegar

1 tablespoon olive oil

**Preparation**
Combine beans, onion and tomato in a large bowl. Add vinegar and oil. Toss to combine. Cover with plastic wrap. Stand for 30 minutes for flavors to develop. Serve.

## Chickpea Capsicum Salad

Serving 4
**List of Ingredients**
1 cup (210g) dried chickpeas

1 1/2 tbs fresh lemon juice

1 tbs extra virgin olive oil

1 garlic clove, peeled, halved

1/2 tsp honey

1/4 tsp smoked paprika

2 red capsicums, quartered, deseeded

1/5 small red onion, halved, thinly sliced

1 bunch continental parsley, leaves picked

1 x 7.10 oz (200g) punnet grape tomatoes, halved

Freshly ground black pepper

**Preparation**
Place chickpeas in a bowl. Cover with cold water and set aside overnight to soak. Drain. Transfer to a saucepan. Cover with cold

water and bring to the boil over high heat. Cook for 35-40 minutes or until tender. Drain. Set aside to cool.

Meanwhile, place the lemon juice, oil, garlic, honey and paprika in a screw-top jar and shake until combined. Set aside for 30 minutes to develop the flavors.

Preheat grill on high. Cook capsicum, skin-side up, under grill for 8-10 minutes or until charred and blistered. Transfer to a heatproof bowl. Cover with plastic wrap and set aside for 10 minutes (this helps lift the skin). Peel skin from the capsicum and cut flesh into thin strips.

Combine chickpeas, capsicum, onion, parsley and tomato in a bowl. Remove garlic from dressing and discard. Drizzle salad with dressing and gently toss to combine. Season with pepper to serve.

## Italian Bean Salad

Serving 4
**List of Ingredients**
1/4 cup olive oil

1 small red onion, diced

2 garlic cloves, crushed

1 celery stalk, finely chopped

1 long red chili, deseeded, finely chopped

14.10 oz (400g) can borlotti beans, drained, rinsed

14.10 oz (400g) can cannellini beans, drained, rinsed

2 roma tomatoes, deseeded, finely chopped

1/4 cup chopped fresh flat-leaf parsley leaves

1 tablespoon red wine vinegar

**Preparation**
Heat oil in a small saucepan over low heat. Add onion, garlic, celery and chili. Cook for 3 minutes or until onion and celery have softened. Stir in beans. Cook for 5 minutes or until heated through. Set aside to cool slightly.

Stir in tomatoes, parsley and vinegar. Season with salt and pepper. Serve.

# Corn Salad

Serving 8
**List of Ingredients**
4 bi-color corn cobs, kernels removed (see note)

1/3 cup chopped fresh coriander leaves

1 small red onion, finely chopped

1 small avocado, finely chopped

8.80 oz (250g) cherry tomatoes, quartered

1/4 cup lime juice

2 tablespoons olive oil

**Preparation**
Bring a saucepan of water to the boil over high heat. Add corn kernels. Cook for 3 to 4 minutes or until corn is tender. Drain. Rinse under cold water.

Combine corn, coriander, onion, avocado, tomatoes, lime juice and oil in a large bowl. Season with salt and pepper. Serve.

## Burghul Salad

Serving 4

**List of Ingredients**

2 red capsicums, halved, deseeded, cut into 4cm pieces

21.20 oz (600g) eggplant, cut into 4cm pieces

2 red onions, halved, cut into thick wedges

1/4 cup (60ml) extra virgin olive oil

1/2 cup (90g) burghul

3/4 cup (185ml) salt-reduced vegetable stock

1 tbs finely grated lemon rind

1/4 cup (60ml) fresh lemon juice

1 bunch coriander, leaves picked, washed, dried

**Preparation**

Preheat oven to 446.00ºF (230°C). Line 2 large roasting pans with non-stick baking paper. Place the capsicum, eggplant and onion in a bowl. Drizzle over the oil. Toss to coat. Transfer to the lined trays. Roast in oven, swapping the trays halfway through cooking, for 40 minutes or until tender and light golden.

Meanwhile, place the burghul in a large heatproof bowl. Bring the stock to the boil in a small saucepan. Pour over the burghul and set aside for 20 minutes or until tender. Drain.

Combine the capsicum mixture and burghul in a bowl.

Add the lemon rind, lemon juice and coriander to the burghul mixture. Season with salt and pepper. Toss to combine. Serve.

# Salad with Eggplant Tomato Parsley and Mint Yoghurt Dressing

Serving 4

**List of Ingredients**

2 (about 10.60 oz or 300g) eggplants, cut into 1cm-thick slices

Olive oil spray

2 ripe tomatoes, finely chopped

1 cup fresh continental parsley leaves

**Mint yoghurt dressing**

1/4 cup (70g) skim milk natural yoghurt

2 tsp bought mint sauce

1 tbs chopped fresh mint

2 tsp fresh lemon juice

**Preparation**

To make dressing, combine the yoghurt, mint sauce, fresh mint and lemon juice in a jug. Season with salt and pepper.

Heat a barbecue grill on high. Lightly spray the eggplant with olive oil spray. Season with salt. Cook for 2 minutes each side or until brown and tender. Cut into 2cm strips.

Place the eggplant, tomato and parsley in a large bowl. Gently toss to combine.

Place the eggplant mixture on a serving plate and drizzle with the dressing. Serve.

# Asparagus Zucchini Salad

Serving 8
**List of Ingredients**
1 1/2 cups fresh broad beans

2 bunches asparagus, trimmed

3 medium zucchini, thinly sliced lengthways

1/4 cup fresh mint leaves

1 teaspoon olive oil

3 teaspoons red wine vinegar

**Preparation**
Place beans in a heatproof bowl. Cover with boiling water. Stand for 3 minutes or until tender. Drain. Refresh under cold water. Drain. Peel.

Heat a barbecue plate or chargrill on medium-high heat. Cook asparagus and zucchini for 2 to 3 minutes each side or until charred and tender. Place asparagus, zucchini, beans and mint in a large bowl.

Place oil and vinegar in a screw-top jar. Secure lid. Shake until combined. Drizzle over asparagus mixture. Season with salt and pepper. Toss to combine. Serve.

# Green Bean Lentil Salad

Serving 4
**List of Ingredients**
8.80 oz (250g) dried brown lentils, rinsed

2 tsp olive oil

1 brown onion, finely chopped

2 garlic cloves, crushed

2 tsp finely grated fresh ginger

2 tsp garam masala

1 tbs fresh lime juice

7.10 oz (200g) green beans, topped

1 x 8.80 oz (250g) punnet cherry tomatoes, quartered

4 celery sticks, ends trimmed, cut into 4cm matchsticks

1/2 cup fresh coriander leaves

1/3 cup (90g) low-fat natural yoghurt, to serve

**Preparation**

Place the lentils and 1.5L (6 cups) cold water in a large saucepan and bring to the boil. Reduce heat to low. Simmer for 25 minutes or until the lentils are just tender. Drain.

Meanwhile, heat the oil in a non-stick frying pan over medium heat. Add the onion and cook, stirring, for 5 minutes or until soft. Add the garlic, ginger and garam masala, and cook, stirring, for 1-2 minutes or until aromatic.

Transfer the onion mixture to a large heatproof bowl. Add the lentils and lime juice, and stir until well combined. Season with pepper. Set aside to cool completely.

Cook the beans in a saucepan of boiling water for 3-4 minutes or until bright green and tender crisp. Refresh under cold running water. Drain. Add the beans, tomato, celery and coriander to the lentil mixture, and stir until just combined. Divide the salad among serving plates. Serve with the yoghurt.

# Lentil Capsicum Salad

Serving 6

**List of Ingredients**

2 tablespoons extra-virgin olive oil

1 tablespoon red wine vinegar

1 baby cos lettuce

14.10 oz (400g) can lentils, drained, rinsed

1 small red capsicum, chopped

1 small avocado, chopped

1/4 red onion, thinly sliced

**Preparation**

Place oil and vinegar in a screw-top jar. Season with salt and pepper. Secure lid. Shake to combine.

Remove outer leaves and core from lettuce. Separate leaves. Wash and pat dry with a tea towel. Roughly chop. Place lettuce, lentils, capsicum, avocado and onion in a bowl. Add dressing. Toss to combine. Serve.

## Lentil Mushrooms Asparagus Salad

Serving 4
**List of Ingredients**
1 x 14.10 oz (400g) can brown lentils, rinsed, and drained

1/2 small red onion, finely chopped

1 tbs balsamic vinegar

Olive oil spray

4 large flat mushrooms, trimmed

2 bunches asparagus, woody ends trimmed, halved crossways

1 large chargrilled red capsicum, cut into thin strips

1/2 cup fresh continental parsley leaves

1/2 cup (125g) low-fat ricotta

Balsamic vinegar, extra, to serve

**Preparation**
Combine the lentils, onion, and vinegar in a large bowl.

Preheat a chargrill on high. Spray with olive oil spray to lightly grease. Cook the mushrooms on grill for 3 minutes each side or until lightly charred and tender. Transfer to a plate. Cook the asparagus on grill for 1-2 minutes each side or until lightly charred and tender crisp.

Add the asparagus, capsicum and parsley to the lentil mixture and toss to combine. Season with pepper.

Halve the mushrooms. Break the ricotta into coarse pieces. Divide the lentil mixture among serving bowls. Top with the mushroom. Drizzle over a little extra vinegar. Top with the ricotta. Season with pepper to serve.

## Chickpea Vegetable Salad

Serving 4
**List of Ingredients**
17.60 oz (500g) small coliban (chat) potatoes

1 bunch asparagus, woody ends trimmed, halved crossways

7.10 oz (200g) sugar snap peas, topped

1 x 14.10 oz (400g) can chickpeas, rinsed, drained

1 large red capsicum, halved, deseeded, cut into 1cm pieces

1 baby cos lettuce, leaves separated, washed, dried

1/2 small red onion, finely chopped

1/4 cup firmly packed finely shredded fresh mint

**Dressing**
2 tsp mild paprika

1 tsp freshly ground black pepper

3/4 tsp ground cumin

3/4 tsp ground coriander

3/4 tsp ground cinnamon

1/2 tsp ground cloves

1/2 tsp ground cardamom

1/2 tsp ground fennel

1 tbs extra virgin olive oil

1 large garlic clove, finely chopped

2 tsp finely grated lemon rind

2 tbs fresh lemon juice

1 tbs water

Salt

**Preparation**

Cook the potatoes in a medium saucepan of boiling water for 15-20 minutes or until tender. Drain. Set aside for 20 minutes to cool.

Cook the asparagus and sugar snap peas in a large saucepan of salted boiling water for 1 minute or until bright green and tender crisp. Drain. Refresh under cold running water. Drain well.

To make the dressing, combine the paprika, pepper, cumin, coriander, cinnamon, cloves, cardamom and fennel in a small bowl. Heat the oil in a small saucepan over medium-low heat. Add the spice mixture and garlic, and cook, stirring, for 30 seconds or until fragrant. Remove from heat. Add the lemon rind, lemon juice and water, and stir to combine. Taste and season with salt.

Cut the potatoes in half crossways and place in a large serving bowl. Add the asparagus, sugar snap peas, chickpeas, capsicum, lettuce, onion and mint. Drizzle with dressing and gently toss to combine. Spoon salad among serving bowls and serve immediately.

## Mustard Green Salad

Serving 6

**List of Ingredients**

3.50 oz (100g) snow peas, trimmed, halved

5.30 oz (150g) sugar snap peas, trimmed

5.30 oz (150g) green beans, trimmed

1/3 cup fresh mint leaves

1.80 oz (50g) baby spinach

1.80 oz (50g) baby rocket

1/3 cup pepitas, toasted

**Mustard dressing**

1 tablespoon olive oil

1 tablespoon red wine vinegar

1 1/2 tablespoons American mustard

**Preparation**

Make dressing Place oil, vinegar and mustard in a screw top jar.

Season with salt and pepper. Secure lid. Refrigerate.

Cook peas and beans in a saucepan of boiling water for 1 to 2 minutes or until just tender. Refresh under cold water. Drain. Place peas and beans, mint, spinach, rocket and pepitas in a bowl or airtight container. Toss to combine. Cover and refrigerate.

# Tomato Asparagus Pasta Salad

Serving 10

**List of Ingredients**

26.50 oz (750g) dried farfalle pasta

4 bunches asparagus, woody ends trimmed, cut into 3cm lengths

14.10 oz (400g) sugar snap peas, trimmed

7.10 oz (200g) punnet yellow grape tomatoes, halved lengthways

7.10 oz (200g) punnet cherry tomatoes, halved

1 cup firmly packed fresh basil leaves, torn

5.30 oz (150g) bocconcini, torn

1/2 cup (80g) pine nuts, lightly toasted

1 tbs finely grated lemon rind

1/4 cup (60ml) fresh lemon juice

2 tbs extra virgin olive oil

1 tbs white balsamic vinegar

**Preparation**

Cook the pasta in a large saucepan of boiling water until al dente. Rinse under cold running water. Drain. Set aside to cool slightly.

Cook the asparagus and sugar snap peas in a saucepan of boiling water for 2 minutes or until bright green and tender crisp. Drain. Place the pasta, asparagus and sugar snap peas in a large bowl.

Add the combined tomato, basil, bocconcini, pine nuts and lemon rind. Whisk the lemon juice, oil, vinegar and sugar in a bowl. Add to the pasta mixture. Toss to combine. Season with pepper.

## Mixed Tomato Salad

Serving 4
**List of Ingredients**
14.10 oz (400g) tomato medley mix

2 small red tomatoes, cut into wedges

1/2 small red onion, finely diced

1 tablespoon extra-virgin olive oil

2 teaspoons red wine vinegar

1/4 cup small fresh basil leaves

**Preparation**
Cut half the medley tomatoes in half. Place in a large shallow dish. Add remaining tomatoes and onion.

Place oil and vinegar in a screw-top jar. Season with salt and pepper. Secure lid. Shake to combine. Add oil mixture to tomato mixture. Gently toss to combine. Set aside at room temperature for 20 minutes for flavors to develop.

Top with basil. Toss to combine. Serve.

# Orange Beetroot Salad

Serving 6
**List of Ingredients**
2 tablespoons extra-virgin olive oil

1 tablespoon orange juice

1 baby cos lettuce

1 large orange, peeled, roughly chopped

15.90 oz (450g) can baby beetroot, drained, and chopped

1 small carrot, peeled, grated

1/4 cup chopped walnuts, toasted

1/4 cup fresh flat-leaf parsley leaves

**Preparation**
Place oil and orange juice in a screw-top jar. Season with salt and pepper. Secure lid. Shake to combine.

Remove outer leaves and core from lettuce. Separate leaves. Wash and pat dry with a tea towel. Roughly chop. Place lettuce, orange, beetroot, carrot, walnuts and parsley in a bowl. Add dressing. Toss to combine. Serve.

# Asparagus Pasta Tomato Salad

Serving 4

**List of Ingredients**

7.10 oz (200g) 8.80 oz dried pasta shapes (such as gnocchi or shells)

8.80 oz (250g) grape tomatoes, quartered lengthways

3 spring onions, finely chopped

1 tbs rice bran oil (See note) or sunflower oil

1 tbs white wine vinegar

2 bunches thin asparagus, woody ends trimmed

**Preparation**

Cook the pasta in a pan of boiling salted water according to packet instructions. Rinse under cold water, then drain well.

Meanwhile, combine the tomatoes, spring onion, oil and vinegar in a large bowl and season to taste with salt and pepper. Leave to stand while the pasta cooks.

Cut the tips from the asparagus. Halve the stems lengthways, then cut into 3cm lengths. Place the tips and stems in a heatproof bowl and pour over enough boiling water to cover. Stand for 1 minute, then rinse under cold water and drain.

Add the asparagus and drained pasta to the tomato mixture, season to taste with salt and pepper, and toss to combine. Divide among serving bowls and serve.

# Bean Pesto Salad

Serving 4
**List of Ingredients**
14.80 oz (420g) can green beans, drained, rinsed

2 x 4.40 oz (125g) cans four bean mix, drained, rinsed

8.80 oz (250g) cherry tomatoes, halved

1/3 cup sundried tomatoes, sliced

1/3 cup kalamata olives, halved

Finely sliced fresh basil leaves, to serve

**Garlic pesto dressing**
2 tablespoons basil pesto

1 garlic clove, crushed

1 tablespoon olive oil

**Preparation**
Make dressing: Place pesto, garlic, oil, and 1 tablespoon cold water in a bowl. Season with salt and pepper. Stir to combine.

Make salad: Place green beans, four bean mix, tomato, sundried tomato and olives in a large bowl.

Season with pepper. Add dressing. Toss to combine. Serve topped with basil.

# Tabouli with Pomegranate

Serving 4

**List of Ingredients**

1/2 cup (90g) burghul

3/4 cup (185ml) boiling water

1 cup chopped fresh continental parsley

3/4 cup chopped fresh mint

2 pomegranates, quartered, seeds removed

3 shallots, trimmed, thinly sliced

2 tbs olive oil

1 tbs fresh lemon juice

**Preparation**

Place the burghul in a large heatproof bowl. Add the boiling water and set aside for 10 minutes to soak. Drain.

Add the parsley, mint, pomegranate seeds, shallot, oil and lemon juice. Season with salt and pepper. Mix until well combined.

## Potato Beetroot Bean Salad

Serving 6
**List of Ingredients**
2.2 lbs (1kg) desiree potatoes, cut into 3cm pieces

2 cups frozen broad beans

15.90 oz (450g) can baby beets, drained, quartered

2 cups watercress sprigs

1 small white onion, thinly sliced

1/4 cup fresh flat-leaf parsley leaves

1/4 cup Praise French dressing

**Preparation**
Cook potato in a large saucepan of boiling, salted water for 8 to 10 minutes or until just tender. Drain. Refresh under cold water. Drain.

Meanwhile, place beans in a heatproof bowl. Cover with boiling water. Stand for 5 minutes or until tender. Drain. Refresh under cold water. Drain. Peel and discard skins. Place beetroot on a plate lined with paper towel. Pat dry.

Place potato, beans, watercress, onion, beetroot and parsley in a bowl. Drizzle with dressing. Toss to combine. Serve.

## Eggplant Chickpea Paprika Yoghurt Salad

Serving 4
**List of Ingredients**
1 large (about 22.90 oz or 650g) eggplant, trimmed, coarsely chopped

2 tsp ground cumin

3 tsp paprika

Olive oil spray

2 x 8.80 oz (250g) punnets cherry tomatoes

1/2 cup (130g) low-fat Greek-style natural yoghurt

1 tbs fresh lemon juice

6 shallots, trimmed, thinly sliced

1 long fresh green chili, seeded, thinly sliced

14.10 oz (400g) can chickpeas, rinsed, and drained

1/4 cup chopped fresh coriander

3.50 oz (100g) baby spinach leaves

## Preparation

Preheat oven to 392.00ºF (200ºC). Line a large baking tray with non-stick baking paper. Place the eggplant, cumin and 2 teaspoons of the paprika in a bowl. Toss to coat. Place the eggplant, in a single layer, on the prepared tray. Spray with oil. Roast for 25 minutes.

Meanwhile, line another baking tray with non-stick baking paper. Place the tomatoes on the tray. Season with pepper and spray with oil. Roast for 12 minutes or until soft.

Combine the yoghurt, lemon juice and remaining paprika in a small bowl.

Combine eggplant, tomatoes, shallot, chili, chickpeas, coriander and spinach in a bowl.

Divide among serving dishes. Serve with the paprika yoghurt.

# Almond Couscous Sultana Salad

Serving 6
**List of Ingredients**
3/4 cup salt-reduced chicken stock

1/2 teaspoon ground cinnamon

3/4 cup couscous

1/2 cup sultanas

1 small red onion, halved, thinly sliced

2 x 14.10 oz (400g) cans chickpeas, drained, rinsed

1/3 cup slivered almonds, toasted

2 tablespoons chopped fresh flat-leaf parsley leaves

1 tablespoon olive oil

**Preparation**
Bring stock and cinnamon to the boil over high heat. Place couscous and sultanas in a large, heatproof bowl. Add stock mixture. Cover. Stand for 3 to 5 minutes or until liquid has absorbed. Stir with a fork to separate grains.

Add onion, chickpeas, almonds, parsley and oil. Season with salt and pepper. Stir to combine. Serve.

## American Style Waldorf Salad

**List of Ingredients**
1 cup red seedless grapes (cut in half)
2 tbsp lemon juice
½ cup low fat mayonnaise
2 finely chopped sticks of celery
4 apples cut into chunky pieces
2 tbsp chopped walnuts

**Preparation**
Place the grapes, celery, apples and walnuts into a salad bowl.
In a separate bowl combine the mayonnaise and lemon juice.
Drizzle your dressing over the salad and toss.

# Brown Rice Vegetable Tofu Salad

Serving 4
**List of Ingredients**
17.60 oz (500g) orange sweet potato, peeled, cut into 2cm pieces

Olive oil cooking spray

1 1/3 cups brown rice

1 corn cob, husks and silks removed

10.60 oz (300g) broccoli, cut into florets

7.10 oz (200g) packet Chinese honey-soy tofu, cut into 2cm cubes

1/3 cup chopped fresh flat-leaf parsley leaves

**Preparation**
Preheat oven to 428.00ºF/392.00ºF (220ºC/200ºC) fan-forced. Place sweet potato on a baking tray lined with baking paper. Spray with oil. Bake for 30 to 35 minutes or until golden and tender.

Meanwhile cook rice according to packet directions. Drain. Rinse. Drain.

Place corn and broccoli in a shallow, microwave-safe bowl. Add 2 tablespoons cold water. Cover with plastic wrap. Microwave on high (100%) for 4 to 5 minutes or until tender. Refresh under cold water. Drain. Cool for 5 minutes. Using a small sharp knife, cut kernels from cob. Cut broccoli into small pieces.

Combine rice, sweet potato, corn, broccoli, tofu and parsley in a bowl. Season with salt and pepper. Serve.

## Club Salad

**List of Ingredients**
1 cup of fat-free salad dressing
2 tbsp chopped onions
2 tbsp shredded chives
¼ tsp salt
½ tsp dry mustard
¼ shredded parsley
¼ cup tarragon vinegar
Pinch of ground black pepper
2 cups chopped lettuce leaves
2 cooked chicken breasts, cubes
2 tomatoes
5 slices of grilled bacon (remove fat before grilling)

**Preparation**
In a medium sized bowl combine the dressing, vinegar, parsley, onions, chives, mustard, salt and pepper. Place in the refrigerator and allow to infuse for a few hours.
Place greens in a salad bowl and cubed chicken pieces right in the centre. Coat the greens and chicken with your dressing and finish off by evenly distributing the slices of tomato and bacon bits.

# Corn, Avo and Brown Rice Salad

**List of Ingredients**
3 cups cooked brown rice
½ cup toasted almonds
1 avocado
2 ears of cooked corn
1 tsp lemon juice
1 tsp canola oil
1 tsp brown rice vinegar
1 tsp tamari soy sauce
4 chopped large lettuce leaves

**Preparation**
Cook rice according to package instructions
Peel the avo and pit before mashing with the cooked rice. Remove the corn from the cob and add to the mixture. Also add the onions and almonds.
In a small bowl combine the oil, vinegar, lemon juice, and tamari sauce. Mix together and pour all over salad. Serve chilled.

# Vegetable Dishes

## Asian Greens Shiitake Mushrooms

Serving 6
**List of Ingredients**
2 tbs olive oil
2 garlic cloves, crushed
2 tsp finely grated fresh ginger
3.50 oz (100g) fresh shiitake mushrooms, thinly sliced
1 bunch baby pak choy, trimmed, leaves separated, stems cut from leaves
1 bunch baby bok choy, trimmed
1 x 15oz (425g) can baby corn spears, drained
2 tbs oyster sauce
1 tbs soy sauce
2 tbs water
**Preparation**
Heat oil in a large frying pan or wok over medium-high heat. Add garlic and ginger. Stir-fry for 30 seconds or until aromatic.
Add the mushroom and stir-fry for 2 minutes. Add the pak choy stems and stir-fry for 1 minute. Add the pak choy leaves, buk choy, corn, oyster sauce and soy sauce. Toss to combine.
Add the water and reduce heat to low. Cover and cook for 2 minutes or until the vegetables are just tender. Serve.

## Roast Vegetables With Balsamic

Serving 8
**List of Ingredients**
4 lbs (1.8kg) Butternut pumpkin, peeled, deseeded, cut into 3cm pieces

6 medium parsnips, peeled, quartered lengthways

2 tbs olive oil

2 bunches baby beetroot, peeled

1 1/2 tbs white balsamic vinegar

16 garlic cloves, unpeeled

1 tbs shredded fresh sage

2 tbs dry-roasted hazelnuts, chopped

**Preparation**
Preheat oven to 392.00ºF (200°C). Line 2 large baking trays with non-stick baking paper.

Place the pumpkin and parsnip in a large bowl. Drizzle over the oil and vinegar. Toss to coat. Arrange on the lined baking trays. Cut the beetroot evenly into quarters. Add the beetroot to the bowl and toss to coat. Add to 1 of the lined baking trays. Sprinkle the garlic around the vegetables. Season with salt and pepper.

Roast, turning once, for 1 hour or until tender. Transfer to a serving dish and sprinkle with the sage and hazelnut.

## Baby Carrots with Honey BBQ

Serving 4
**List of Ingredients**
2 bunches baby (Dutch) carrots, trimmed

1 tablespoon olive oil

1 tablespoon honey

8 garlic cloves, unpeeled

**Preparation**
Preheat a covered barbecue on medium-high heat with hood down. Combine carrots, oil, honey and garlic in a large foil baking tray. Season with salt and pepper. Toss to combine.

Barbecue, with hood down, using indirect heat (see note), for 15 to 20 minutes, turning halfway during cooking time, or until carrots are caramelized and just tender. Serve.

# Mushrooms Asparagus BBQ

Serving 8
**List of Ingredients**
8 flat mushrooms

2 bunches asparagus, trimmed

Olive oil cooking spray

2 tablespoons extra-virgin olive oil

1 tablespoon lemon juice

**Preparation**

Preheat a barbecue or chargrill on medium-high heat. Spray mushrooms and asparagus with oil. Cook for 2 minutes each side or until just tender.

Place vegetables on a large plate. Drizzle with oil and lemon juice. Season with salt and pepper. Serve.

# Mushrooms Cajun Style

Serving 4
**List of Ingredients**
1 tablespoon olive oil

17.60 oz (500g) cup mushrooms, quartered

1/2 teaspoon dried chili flakes

2 garlic cloves, crushed

2 teaspoons dried oregano

Pinch ground turmeric

**Preparation**
Heat oil in a large frying pan over high heat. Add mushroom. Cook, stirring, for 5 minutes or until golden and tender.

Add chili, garlic, oregano and turmeric. Cook, stirring, for 1 minute or until fragrant. Season with salt and pepper. Serve.

# Curried Cauliflower, Chickpea, Coriander Tomato

Serving 4

**List of Ingredients**

Olive oil spray

1 red onion, halved, cut into thin wedges

2 garlic cloves, crushed

2 long fresh green chilies, halved, deseeded, finely chopped

1 tsp cumin seeds, lightly crushed (see tip)

2 tsp ground coriander

1/2 tsp ground turmeric

2 x 8.80 oz (250g) punnets cherry tomatoes, halved

17.60 oz (500g) cauliflower, trimmed, cut into florets

1/2 cup (125ml) water

1 x 14.10 oz (400g) can chickpeas, rinsed, drained

7.10 oz (200g) green beans, topped, cut into 3cm lengths

2 tbs chopped fresh coriander

Steamed basmati rice, to serve

Fresh coriander leaves, to serve

## Preparation

Spray a wok or large non-stick frying pan lightly with olive oil spray. Heat over medium-high heat. Add the onion and stir-fry for 3 minutes or until light golden. Add the garlic, chili, cumin seeds, ground coriander and turmeric. Stir-fry for 1 minute or until aromatic.

Stir in the tomato, cauliflower and water. Bring to the boil. Reduce heat to low. Simmer, covered, for 6 minutes.

Stir in the chickpeas and beans. Simmer, covered, for 3 minutes or until beans are bright green and tender crisp.

Stir in the chopped coriander and season with pepper. Divide the rice and curry among serving bowls. Top with coriander leaves to serve.

## Couscous Chickpea Capsicum

Serving 4
**List of Ingredients**
2 large 21.20 oz (600g) red capsicums, halved, deseeded
3 tsp olive oil
2/3 cup (140g) couscous
1 1/4 cups (310ml) boiling water
1 brown onion, chopped
1 10.60 oz (300g) can chickpeas, rinsed, drained
1/2 cup (85g) chopped dried pitted dates
1/2 tsp ground ginger
1/4 tsp cayenne pepper
1/4 tsp salt
1/3 cup loosely packed chopped fresh continental parsley
1 7.10 oz (200g) container natural set yoghurt, 99.8% fat free

**Preparation**
Preheat oven to 428.00ºF (220°C). Brush capsicums with 1 tsp of oil. Place, cut-side up, in roasting pan lined with foil. Roast for 10 minutes or until tender.

Meanwhile, place couscous in a heatproof bowl and pour over boiling water, stirring with a fork. Cover, set aside for 5 minutes or until liquid is absorbed. Fluff with fork. Heat remaining oil in a non-stick frying pan over high heat. Cook onion, stirring, for 5-6 minutes or until brown. Reduce heat to medium, add couscous, chickpeas, dates, ginger, pepper and salt. Cook, stirring, for 2-3 minutes or until combined. Add parsley.

Remove capsicum from oven. Spoon couscous mixture into each half. Bake for 12-15 minutes or until brown. Serve with the yoghurt.

# Chickpea Veggie Burgers

Serving 4

**List of Ingredients**

14.10 oz (400g) can chickpeas, drained, rinsed

1 small (2.50 oz or 70g) carrot, peeled, grated

2/3 cup wholegrain breadcrumbs

2 eggs, lightly beaten

2 teaspoons olive oil

4 round wholegrain rolls, halved crossways

8 green oak lettuce leaves

4 slices canned beetroot, drained

1 large (7.80 oz or 220g) tomato, sliced

**Preparation**

Place chickpeas in a bowl. Using a fork, mash until almost smooth. Add carrot, breadcrumbs and egg. Mix to combine. Using floured hands, shape mixture into 4 patties.

Heat oil in a frying pan over medium heat. Cook patties, turning, for 4 to 5 minutes each side or until heated through.

Meanwhile, preheat grill on high. Toast cut side of rolls for 2 to 3 minutes or until golden. Top roll bases with beetroot, lettuce, tomato, patties and roll tops. Serve.

# Sweet Potato Fennel Chili

Serving 4
**List of Ingredients**
28.20 oz (800g) small orange sweet potato, unpeeled

2 tablespoons vegetable oil

1 1/2 tablespoons plain flour

1/2 teaspoon dried chili flakes, finely crushed

1 teaspoon fennel seeds, finely crushed

1 teaspoon sea salt

**Preparation**
Preheat oven to 428.00ºF/392.00ºF (220ºC/200ºC) fan-forced. Cut potato into 1.5cm-thick slices. Place potato in a large saucepan. Cover with cold water. Bring to the boil over high heat. Reduce heat to medium. Boil for 3 minutes or until almost tender. Drain.

Return potato to saucepan over low heat. Cook, shaking pan, for 30 seconds or until potato is dry. Transfer to a baking paper-lined baking tray. Drizzle with oil. Cool for 10 minutes. Combine flour, chili, fennel and salt in a small bowl. Sprinkle flour mixture over potato. Toss to coat. Spread potato, in a single layer, over tray.

Bake for 40 minutes, turning potato halfway through cooking, or until golden and crisp.

## Spicy Couscous and Sunflower Seeds

Serving 4

**List of List of Ingredients**

1 1/2 cups couscous

1 1/2 cups boiling water

1 tablespoon olive oil

1 teaspoon ground fennel seeds

1 teaspoon ground cumin

1/2 teaspoon ground turmeric

1/3 cup sunflower seeds

1 long red chili, deseeded, thinly sliced

2.10 oz (60g) baby rocket

3.50 oz (100g) cherry tomatoes, halved

**Preparation**

Place couscous and boiling water in a large, heatproof bowl. Stand, covered, for 4 to 5 minutes or until water is absorbed. Stir with a fork to separate grains.

Meanwhile, heat oil in a large frying pan over medium-low heat. Add fennel, cumin, turmeric and sunflower seeds. Cook, stirring, for 2 to 3 minutes or until seeds are coated. Remove from heat.

Add chili, rocket, tomato and couscous to pan. Gently toss to combine. Serve.

# Curried Lentil Pumpkin

Serving 6
**List of Ingredients**
1 tbs vegetable oil

2 brown onions, finely chopped

3 garlic cloves, peeled, thinly sliced lengthways

2 x 7cm cinnamon sticks

3 large fresh green chilies, thickly sliced

1 tbs black mustard seeds

3 tsp ground cumin

3 tsp ground turmeric

17.60 oz (500g) butternut pumpkin, peeled, deseeded, cut into 4cm pieces

1 1/2 cups (305g) dried brown or green lentils

5 cups (1.25L) vegetable stock

3 celery stalks, including leaves, coarsely chopped

Salt & freshly ground black pepper

Steamed basmati rice, to serve.

**Preparation**

Heat oil in a large saucepan over medium-low heat. Add onion and garlic and cook, stirring, for 10 minutes or until soft. Add the cinnamon, chili, mustard seeds, cumin and turmeric and cook, stirring, for 1 minute or until aromatic.

Add pumpkin, lentils and stock to onion mixture. Increase heat to medium and bring to the boil. Reduce heat to medium-low and cook, covered, for 20 minutes. Add celery. Cook for 10 minutes or until lentils are tender. Season with salt and pepper.

Divide curry among serving bowls. Serve with steamed basmati rice.

# Curried Wraps with Vegetable Couscous

Serving 4
**List of Ingredients**
2 teaspoons olive oil

1 red capsicum, chopped

1 garlic clove, crushed

1 tablespoon ground cumin

1 tablespoon ground coriander

1 teaspoon ground turmeric

7.10 oz (200g) baby eggplant, chopped

10.60 oz (300g) zucchini, chopped

10.60 oz (300g) tomatoes, chopped

1 cup couscous

1 cup boiling water

4 pieces mountain bread

Lemon wedges and mint yoghurt, to serve

## Preparation

Heat oil in a frying pan over medium-high heat. Add capsicum, garlic, cumin, coriander and turmeric. Cook, stirring, for 1 minute or until fragrant. Add eggplant and zucchini. Cook, stirring, for 5 minutes or until browned. Add tomatoes. Cook, covered, for 5 minutes or until vegetables soften.

Meanwhile, place couscous in a heatproof bowl. Pour over boiling water. Cover. Stand for 5 minutes or until liquid is absorbed. Stir with a fork to separate grains.

Add vegetable mixture to couscous. Stir to combine. Place bread on plates. Top with mixture. Roll up tightly to enclose filling. Serve with lemon wedges and mint yoghurt.

# Falafel

Serving 4

**List of Ingredients**

1 brown onion, chopped

2 garlic cloves, chopped

2 teaspoons ground coriander

1 teaspoon cumin seeds

2 x 400g cans chickpeas, drained, rinsed

1 cup chopped fresh flat-leaf parsley leaves

1/3 cup plain flour

1 egg white

1 tablespoon olive oil

Tabouli, yoghurt and lavash bread, to serve

**Preparation**

Place onion, garlic, coriander, cumin, chickpeas, parsley, flour, egg white, salt and pepper in a food processor. Process until almost smooth. Using floured hands, shape mixture into four 2cm-thick patties. Place on a plate. Cover and refrigerate for 30 minutes.

Heat oil in a large frying pan over medium heat. Cook patties for 4 to 5 minutes each side or until cooked through.

Serve with tabouli, yoghurt and bread.

## Falafel Hummus Wrap

Serving 4

**List of Ingredients**

4 multigrain wraps

1/2 cup hummus dip

1/2 baby cos lettuce, leaves separated, torn

5.30 oz (150g) tabouli

1 Lebanese cucumber, cut into ribbons

6 (225g) falafel with sesame seeds, halved

**Preparation**

Place wraps on a flat surface.
Spread hummus along centre of each wrap.
Top with lettuce, tabouli, cucumber and 3 falafel halves.
Roll up firmly to enclose filling. Serve.

# Spice Vegetable Stir-Fry

Serving 4
**List of Ingredients**
1 1/2 tsp cornflour

2 tbs light soy sauce

2 tbs Chinese rice wine (shaohsing)* or dry sherry

2 tsp five-spice powder

1 tbs vegetable oil

2 red capsicums, thinly sliced

1 yellow capsicum, thinly sliced

2 bunches broccolini, trimmed, halved on the diagonal

7.10 oz (200g) fresh shiitake mushrooms*, thinly sliced

1 1/4 cups (275g) medium-grain white rice, steamed, to serve

**Preparation**
Combine cornflour and 1/3 cup (80ml) cold water in a bowl. Add soy sauce, Chinese rice wine, and five-spice, and mix well. Meanwhile, heat the oil in a wok over high heat until smoking.

Add the vegetables and stir-fry for 2 minutes. Add sauce mixture and stir-fry for 2 minutes or until vegetables have softened but are still crunchy, and sauce has thickened.

Divide the stir-fry among serving plates and serve with steamed rice.

# Garlic Thyme Mushrooms

Serving 4
**List of Ingredients**
14.10 oz (400g) button mushrooms

7.10 oz (200g) Swiss brown mushrooms, halved

2 garlic cloves, thinly sliced

1 tablespoon fresh thyme leaves

2 tablespoons olive oil

1.80 oz (50g) reduced-fat feta cheese, crumbled

**Preparation**
Preheat oven to 392.00ºF/356.00ºF (200°C/180°C) fan-forced. Place mushroom, garlic, and thyme in a large baking dish. Drizzle with oil. Toss to combine.

Bake, stirring halfway through cooking, for 20 to 25 minutes or until mushrooms are tender and browned.

Season with salt and pepper. Top with feta. Serve.

# Tofu Ginger Mushrooms

Serving 6

**List of Ingredients**

1 tablespoon vegetable oil

1 brown onion, thinly sliced

2 garlic cloves, sliced

4cm piece fresh ginger, peeled, cut into thin matchsticks

600g firm tofu, cut into 3cm squares

200g Swiss brown mushrooms, halved

100g enoki mushrooms, trimmed

2 tablespoons light soy sauce

1/3 cup vegetarian stir-fry sauce (see note)

1 bunch gai lan (Chinese broccoli), chopped

440g packet udon noodles

**Preparation**

Heat oil in a wok over medium-high heat. Stir-fry onion and garlic for 2 to 3 minutes or until just soft. Add ginger and tofu. Stir-fry for 3 minutes.

Add mushrooms, soy sauce and stir-fry sauce. Stir-fry for 2 minutes. Add gai lan. Stir-fry 1 to 2 minutes or until gai lan is just tender. Remove from heat.

Place noodles in a heatproof bowl. Cover with boiling water. Set aside for 2 to 3 minutes or until heated through. Use a fork, separate noodles. Drain. Serve noodles with ginger tofu and mushrooms.

# Chickpea Sweet Potato Patties

Serving 4

**List of Ingredients**

17.60 oz (500g) kumara (orange sweet potato), peeled, cut into 2cm pieces

14.80 oz (420g) can chickpeas, drained, rinsed

1/3 cup couscous

1 teaspoon garam masala

2 garlic cloves, crushed

1 egg, lightly beaten

3 teaspoons olive oil

1/2 cup low-fat natural yoghurt

2 tablespoons mango chutney

2.10 oz (60g) salad leaves, to serve

**Preparation**

Place kumara onto a microwave-safe plate in a single layer. Cover. Microwave for 3 to 5 minutes on HIGH (100%) power or until just tender. Drain. Transfer to a bowl. Add chickpeas. Mash mixture until almost smooth.

Add couscous, garam masala, garlic, egg, and salt to kumara mixture. Mix until well combined. Using damp hands, form mixture into 8 x 1.5cm-thick patties.

Heat oil in a large non-stick frying pan over medium heat. Cook patties for 3 to 4 minutes each side or until golden and heated through.

Combine yoghurt and chutney in a small bowl. Serve patties with mango yoghurt and salad leaves.

# Roast Tomato on Lentil Patties

Serving 4

**List of Ingredients**

8.80 oz (250g) punnet cherry tomatoes, halved

1/3 cup basil, finely shredded

17.60 oz (500g) sweet potato, peeled, cut into 3cm pieces

2 teaspoons olive oil

1 small onion, finely chopped

1 garlic clove, crushed

1 teaspoon ground cumin

1 teaspoon ground coriander

2 x 14.10 oz (400g) cans brown lentils, rinsed, drained

1/3 cup packaged breadcrumbs

1/3 cup vegetable oil, for cooking

Baby rocket leaves dressed with lemon juice, to serve

**Preparation**

Preheat oven to 356.00ºF (180°C). Arrange tomatoes, cut side up, on an oven tray. Roast for 30 minutes or until soft and lightly browned. Cool for 15 minutes. Transfer to a food processor and process to form a chunky sauce. Season with pepper. Stir in half the basil.

Wash sweet potato. Place on a microwave-safe, heatproof plate. Cover and cook for 5 minutes on HIGH (100%) or until tender. Drain. Transfer sweet potato to a bowl. Mash roughly with a fork.

Heat oil in a saucepan over medium heat. Add onion and cook for 5 minutes or until light golden. Add garlic, cumin and coriander and cook, stirring, for 1 minute.

Using a fork, combine sweet potato, onion mixture, lentils and salt and pepper. Shape into 8 patties. Coat both sides lightly with breadcrumbs.

Heat oil in a frying pan over medium heat. Cook patties, in batches, for 2 minutes each side or until golden. Place patties on plates. Spoon over sauce. Top with remaining basil. Serve with rocket.

# Chili Con Carne

Serving 4
**List of Ingredients**
1 tablespoon olive oil

1 medium brown onion, finely chopped

2 garlic cloves, crushed

17.60 oz (500g) lean beef mince

2 teaspoons ground cumin

2 teaspoons ground coriander

1 teaspoon cayenne pepper

2 tablespoons tomato paste

1 medium carrot, peeled, grated

1 medium zucchini, grated

14.10 oz (400g) can chopped tomatoes

14.80 oz (420g) can kidney beans, drained, rinsed

7.10 oz (200g) tub 99.8% fat-free plain yoghurt

4 cups cooked doongara rice, to serve

**Preparation**

Heat oil in a large deep frying pan over medium-high heat. Cook onion, stirring, for 5 minutes or until softened. Add garlic. Cook, stirring, for 1 minute or until fragrant.

Add mince. Cook, stirring with a wooden spoon to break up mince, for 5 minutes or until browned. Add cumin, coriander and cayenne pepper. Cook for 30 seconds or until fragrant. Add tomato paste. Cook, stirring, for 30 seconds. Add carrot and zucchini. Stir until coated. Add tomatoes and beans. Cover. Reduce heat to low. Simmer, stirring occasionally, for 30 minutes or until thickened.

Serve with yoghurt and rice.

# Zucchini White Beans Cherry Tomatoes

Serving 4

**List of Ingredients**

1 tablespoon olive oil

1 medium red onion, halved, sliced

2 garlic cloves, thinly sliced

1 tablespoon mild paprika

8.80 oz (250g) cherry tomatoes, halved

1 medium zucchini, thinly sliced

14.80 oz (420g) can cannellini beans, drained, rinsed

1 teaspoon balsamic vinegar

1/2 cup fresh flat leaf parsley leaves, chopped

2.80 oz (80g) baby rocket

4 slices wholegrain low-GI bread, toasted, to serve

**Preparation**

Heat oil in a large frying pan over medium heat. Cook onion, stirring, for 5 minutes or until softened. Add garlic. Cook, stirring, for 1 minute. Add paprika. Cook for 30 seconds or until fragrant.

Add tomatoes and zucchini. Cook for 3 to 4 minutes or until tomatoes start to collapse. Add beans and vinegar. Cook for 5 minutes or until heated through. Stir in parsley. Season with pepper. Serve with rocket and bread.

## Artichokes Marinated

Serving 6

**List of Ingredients**

2 x 14.10 oz (400g) cans artichoke hearts, drained, halved

3 thick strips lemon rind

2 small red chilies, deseeded, thinly sliced

2 tablespoons white wine vinegar

1/4 cup extra-virgin olive oil

2 tablespoons coarsely chopped fresh flat-leaf parsley leaves

2 garlic cloves, halved, thinly sliced

**Preparation**

Pat artichokes dry with paper towel. Combine artichokes, lemon rind, chili, vinegar, oil, parsley and garlic in a glass or ceramic bowl. Cover. Refrigerate for at least 2 days for flavors to develop, stirring twice each day.

## Stir Fry Tofu Shiitake Mushrooms

Serving 4
**List of Ingredients**
10.60 oz (300g) firm tofu, cut into thin strips

1/4 cup (60ml) mirin (rice wine)

2 tbs salt-reduced soy sauce

2 tsp finely grated fresh ginger

1 tsp brown sugar

Vegetable oil spray

1 red onion, cut into thin wedges

5.30 oz (150g) shiitake mushrooms, halved

2 bunches broccolini, ends trimmed, cut into 2cm lengths

1 red capsicum, deseeded, thinly sliced

1 tsp sesame seeds

Steamed basmati rice, to serve

## Preparation

Place the tofu in a shallow glass or ceramic dish. Combine half the mirin, soy sauce and ginger in a jug and pour over the tofu. Cover with plastic wrap and place in the fridge for 30 minutes to marinate.

Combine the sugar and remaining mirin, soy sauce and ginger in a small bowl. Heat a wok or frying pan over high heat. Lightly spray with olive oil spray. Drain the tofu and reserve the marinade. Add one-third of the tofu to the wok and cook for 1-2 minutes each side or until golden brown. Transfer to a plate. Repeat, in 2 more batches, with the remaining tofu.

Lightly spray the wok with olive oil spray. Add the onion and stir-fry for 1 minute or until brown. Add the mushroom and stir-fry for 1-2 minutes or until tender. Add the broccolini and capsicum and stir-fry for 1 minute or until almost tender. Add the tofu, mirin mixture and reserved marinade and stir-fry for 1-2 minutes or until broccolini is tender crisp and the marinade comes to the boil.

Divide the rice among serving bowls. Top with the stir-fry and sprinkle with sesame seeds to serve.

# Mexican Beans on Rice

Serving 4
**List of Ingredients**
Olive oil spray

1 brown onion, finely chopped

2 celery sticks, trimmed, finely chopped

1 large carrot, peeled, finely chopped

2 garlic cloves, crushed

1 long fresh red chili, finely chopped

1 tsp ground cumin

1 tsp paprika

1 x 14.10 oz (400g) can no-added-salt diced tomatoes

1 x (400g) can four bean mix, rinsed, drained

3/4 cup (185ml) water

1 red capsicum, halved, deseeded, finely chopped

2 tbs chopped fresh coriander

Steamed rice, to serve

1/3 cup (80ml) low-fat natural yoghurt

Chopped fresh coriander, extra, to serve

### Preparation

Heat a large non-stick frying pan over medium-low heat. Spray with olive oil spray. Add the onion, celery and carrot. Cook, stirring occasionally, for 6-7 minutes.

Add the garlic, chili, cumin and paprika. Cook, stirring, for 1-2 minutes.

Stir in the tomato, beans and water. Increase heat to high. Bring to the boil. Reduce heat to low. Simmer, stirring often, for 10 minutes. Add capsicum and cook for 5 minutes or until the mixture thickens.

Stir in coriander. Divide rice and bean mixture among serving bowls. Top with yoghurt and extra coriander to serve.

# Ratatouille

Serving 6
**List of Ingredients**
1/4 cup (60ml) extra virgin olive oil

1 (about 14.10 oz or 400g) eggplant, cut into 4cm pieces

2 zucchini, trimmed, halved lengthways, coarsely chopped

2 red onions, halved, cut into wedges

1 red capsicum, halved, seeded, cut into 4cm pieces

1 yellow capsicum, halved, seeded, cut into 4cm pieces

3 garlic cloves, finely chopped

1 tbs chopped fresh rosemary

6 (about 22.90 oz or 650g) roma tomatoes, quartered

1/4 cup chopped fresh continental parsley

**Preparation**
Preheat oven to 392.00ºF (200ºC). Heat the oil in a large baking dish in oven for 5 minutes. Stir in the eggplant, zucchini, onion, combined capsicum, garlic and rosemary to coat. Top with tomato.

Bake for 45 minutes or until the vegetables are tender. Stir in the parsley.

# Chickpea Pumpkin Burger

Serving 1
**List of Ingredients**
2 tsp olive oil

1 wholegrain bread roll, split

1 1/2 tbs sweet chili sauce (optional)

Baby spinach leaves, to serve

1/4 small red onion, very thinly sliced

**Pumpkin & chickpea patty**
4.60 oz (130g) Kent pumpkin, peeled, deseeded, cut into 2cm pieces

1 x 4.40 oz (125g) can Edgell chickpeas, rinsed, drained, coarsely mashed

1 1/2 tbs fresh wholegrain breadcrumbs (made from day-old wholegrain bread)

1 tbs dry-roasted walnuts, coarsely chopped

2 tsp chopped fresh chives

1 egg white, lightly whisked

1/2 tsp finely grated lemon rind

## Preparation

To make the pumpkin & chickpea patty, cook the pumpkin in a medium saucepan of boiling water for 3 minutes or until almost tender. Drain. Transfer to a bowl and use a potato masher to coarsely mash. Add the chickpeas, breadcrumbs, walnut, chives, egg white and lemon rind. Season with salt and pepper. Use your hands to mix until combined. Shape into a 2.5cm-thick, 9cm-diameter patty. Place on a plate. Cover with plastic wrap and place in the fridge for 30 minutes to chill.

Heat the oil in a small non-stick frying pan over medium heat. Cook the patty for 4 minutes each side or until heated through.

Meanwhile, preheat grill on high. Place the roll, cut-side up, on a baking tray. Cook under grill for 2 minutes or until toasted.

Place the bread roll base on a serving plate. Spread with half the sweet chili sauce, if desired. Top with the pumpkin & chickpea patty, spinach and onion. Top with remaining bread roll and serve, with the remaining sweet chili sauce if desired.

# Spinach Lentil Dhal

Serving 4
**List of Ingredients**
1 tablespoon peanut oil

2 medium brown onions, thinly sliced

1 garlic clove, crushed

1 tablespoon ground coriander

1 teaspoon ground cumin

1 teaspoon ground turmeric

2 cups red lentils

14.10 oz (400g) can crushed tomatoes

1.80 oz (50g) baby spinach, trimmed, chopped

1/3 cup fresh coriander leaves

4 chapati breads, warmed (see note)

**Preparation**

Heat oil in a saucepan over medium heat. Add onion. Cook, stirring, for 5 minutes or until soft. Add garlic, coriander, cumin and turmeric. Cook, stirring, for 1 minute or until fragrant.

Add lentils, tomato and 2 1/2 cups cold water. Cover. Bring to the boil. Reduce heat to low. Simmer, stirring occasionally, for 20 minutes or until lentils are tender. Add spinach. Cook, stirring, for 2 minutes or until spinach is wilted.

Top lentil mixture with coriander. Season with pepper. Serve with chapati bread.

## Spicy Chickpea Vegetable Soup

Serving 4
**List of Ingredients**
1 tbs olive oil

1 x 14.10 oz (400g) pkt fresh veggie mix

1 tbs finely grated fresh ginger

1 garlic clove, crushed

2 tsp hot curry powder

1 tsp ground cumin

1L (4 cups) water

2 x 14.10 oz (400g) cans Edgell chickpeas, rinsed, drained

1 x 14.10 oz (400g) can diced tomatoes

1/3 cup (90g) low-fat natural yoghurt

1/3 cup small fresh mint leaves

**Preparation**
Heat the oil in a large saucepan over medium heat. Add the vegetable mixture and cook for 3 minutes or until soft.

Add the ginger, garlic, curry powder and cumin to the vegetables. Stir to coat.

Add the water, chickpeas and tomato to the pan. Bring to the boil. Reduce heat to medium. Simmer for 10 minutes. Season with salt and pepper.

Ladle the soup among serving bowls. Top with yoghurt and mint to serve.

## Parcels of Spiced Pumpkin & Chickpea

Serving 4
**List of Ingredients**
2 tsp peanut oil

1 tsp brown mustard seeds

1 tsp ground cumin

1 tsp ground coriander

1 tsp garam masala

1/2 tsp ground turmeric

17.60 oz (500g) butternut pumpkin, cut into 3cm pieces

1 x 14.10 oz (400g) can chickpeas, rinsed, drained

1 brown onion, halved, coarsely chopped

12 fresh curry leaves

Salt & freshly ground black pepper

1 cup (200g) basmati rice

1 1/2 cups (375ml) chicken or vegetable stock

1 Lebanese cucumber, finely chopped

3/4 cup (200g) skim milk natural yoghurt

**Preparation**
Preheat oven to 392.00ºF (200°C). Heat the oil in a small frying pan over medium heat. Add the mustard seeds, cumin, coriander, garam masala and turmeric, and cook, stirring, for 1 minute or until seeds pop and mixture is fragrant. Remove from heat.

Place the pumpkin, chickpeas, onion and curry leaves in a large bowl. Add the spice mixture and season with salt and pepper. Gently toss to coat pumpkin in spice mixture. Combine rice and 125ml (1/2 cup) of stock in a medium bowl.

Cut four 40cm-square pieces of foil and four 40cm-square pieces of nonstick baking paper. Place foil on a clean work surface. Top with the baking paper. Spoon rice mixture evenly among squares. Top with pumpkin mixture and drizzle with the remaining stock.

Fold the foil and paper in half to enclose the fillings. Fold the edges over to seal the parcels. Place parcels on 2 baking trays.

Bake in preheated oven, swapping trays halfway through cooking, for 30 minutes or until pumpkin and rice are tender. Remove from oven. Set aside for 5 minutes to cool slightly.

Meanwhile, combine cucumber and yoghurt in a small bowl. Season with salt and pepper. Carefully transfer contents of parcels to serving bowls. Top with yoghurt mixture and serve immediately.

# Eggplant with Spicy Rice

Serving 4
**List of Ingredients**
3/4 cup (150g) basmati rice

2 large eggplants

1 tbs olive oil

1 large brown onion, halved, finely chopped

1 red capsicum, halved, deseeded, finely chopped

2 garlic cloves, crushed

2 tsp ground coriander

1 tsp finely grated fresh ginger

1/5 tsp finely chopped fresh red chili

1/4 tsp ground turmeric

1/5 cup coarsely chopped fresh continental parsley

2 tsp finely grated lemon rind

2 tbs fresh lemon juice

1/2 cup (130g) reduced-fat yoghurt

2 tbs coarsely chopped fresh mint

**Preparation**
Preheat oven to 392.00ºF (200°C). Cook the rice in a large saucepan of boiling water for 15 minutes or until tender. Rinse under cold running water. Drain well.

Meanwhile, cut the eggplants in half lengthways. Use a small sharp knife to cut a 1cm border around the edge of each eggplant half. Scoop out the flesh within the border, leaving about 1.5cm of flesh on the base of each eggplant half. Finely chop the flesh.

Heat oil in a frying pan over medium heat. Add the onion and capsicum and cook, stirring, for 5 minutes or until soft. Add the garlic, coriander, ginger, chili and turmeric and cook, stirring, for 30 seconds or until aromatic. Add the chopped eggplant and cook, stirring, for 10 minutes or until eggplant is soft. Remove from heat.

Add the rice, parsley, lemon rind and lemon juice to eggplant mixture, and stir to combine. Place eggplant shells in a large baking dish. Spoon rice mixture evenly among eggplant shells. Bake in oven for 30 minutes or until eggplant shells are soft and filling is golden.

Place the yoghurt and mint in a small serving bowl and stir to combine. Serve with spicy rice-filled eggplant.

## Noodles Tofu Pak Choy

Serving 4
**List of Ingredients**
14.10 oz (400g) fresh rice noodles

2 tsp olive oil

1 brown onion, halved, thinly sliced

1 garlic clove, thinly sliced

1 carrot, peeled, thinly sliced

1 red capsicum, halved, deseeded, thinly sliced

8 small cup mushrooms, thickly sliced

1/4 cup (60ml) hoisin sauce

2 tbs kecap manis

10.60 oz (300g) firm tofu, coarsely chopped

1 bunch baby pak choy, trimmed, leaves separated

**Preparation**
Place the noodles in a large heatproof bowl. Cover with boiling water. Set aside for 5 minutes or until soft. Drain.

Meanwhile, heat a wok or large frying pan over high heat. Heat the oil until smoking. Stir-fry the onion and garlic for 3 minutes or until the onion is soft. Add the carrot, capsicum and mushroom. Stir-fry for 3 minutes or until just tender.

Add the noodles, hoisin sauce, kecap manis and tofu to the wok. Stir-fry for 2 minutes or until heated through. Add the pak choy and stir-fry for 1 minute or until pak choy just wilts.

# Sweet Chili Vegetable Burger

Serving 4
**List of Ingredients**
14.10 oz (400g) orange sweet potato, peeled, roughly chopped

1 small carrot, peeled, grated

1 small zucchini, grated

1/4 cup frozen corn kernels, thawed

1/4 cup frozen peas, thawed

2 green onions, chopped

1 egg, lightly beaten

1/2 cup plain flour

2 teaspoons olive oil

4 multigrain bread rolls, halved

1.80 oz (50g) baby spinach

2 tablespoons Fountain sweet chili sauce

## Preparation

Cook sweet potato in a saucepan of boiling, salted water for 8 to 10 minutes or until just tender. Drain. Refresh under cold water. Transfer to a bowl. Mash.

Add carrot, zucchini, corn, peas, onion, egg and flour. Stir to combine. Shape mixture into four 2cm-thick patties.

Heat oil in a non-stick frying pan over medium-high heat. Cook patties for 4 to 5 minutes each side or until golden and cooked through.

Place patties on roll bases. Top with spinach, sauce and roll tops. Serve.

# Tomato Hummus Breadstick

Serving 4

**List of Ingredients**

30cm baguette (French breadstick)

1 garlic clove, peeled, halved

2 ripe tomatoes, finely chopped

2 tbs shredded fresh basil

1/3 cup (90g) hummus

**Preparation**

Preheat a grill on medium-high. Cut a 30cm baguette (French breadstick) diagonally into 2cm-thick slices. Place the bread slices, in a single layer, on a baking tray. Cook under grill for 1-2 minutes each side or until toasted. Rub 1 garlic clove, peeled, halved, over 1 side of each piece of toast. Combine 2 ripe tomatoes, finely chopped, and 2 tbs shredded fresh basil in a small bowl. Spread the toasts evenly with 1/3 cup (90g) hummus. Top with the tomato mixture and serve immediately.

# Quinoa Vegetable Pilaf

Serving 8
**List of Ingredients**
4 cups salt-reduced vegetable stock

2 cups (350g) quinoa (see note)

Olive oil cooking spray

2 medium red capsicums, roughly chopped

1 medium eggplant, roughly chopped

2 medium zucchini, roughly chopped

4 green onions, thinly sliced

2 tablespoons fresh oregano leaves

1/3 cup lemon juice

Fresh oregano leaves, to serve

**Preparation**
Place stock and quinoa in a large saucepan over medium-high heat. Bring to the boil. Reduce heat to low. Simmer covered,

stirring occasionally, for 10 minutes or until just tender. Remove from heat. Set aside, covered for 10 minutes.

Spray a heavy-based saucepan with oil. Heat over medium-high heat. Add capsicum and eggplant. Cook, stirring, for 1 to 2 minutes or until beginning to soften. Cook, covered, for 15 minutes or until softened. Add zucchini, onion and oregano. Toss to combine. Cook, covered, for 5 minutes or until zucchini is tender.

Add zucchini mixture and lemon juice to quinoa. Toss to combine. Season with pepper. Sprinkle with oregano.

## Apricot Vegetables

Serving 4
**List of Ingredients**
2 tsp olive oil

1 brown onion, halved, cut into wedges

2 carrots, peeled, coarsely chopped

2 garlic cloves, crushed

2 tsp finely grated fresh ginger

2 tsp cumin seeds

2 tsp ground paprika

1 x 7cm cinnamon stick

Large pinch of saffron threads

1 1/2 cups (375ml) vegetable stock

22.90 oz (650g) butternut pumpkin, deseeded, peeled, coarsely chopped

8.80 oz (250g) green beans, topped, cut into 6cm lengths

3.50 oz (100g) dried Turkish apricots

3.50 oz (100g) fresh dates, halved, pitted

1 x 14.10 oz (400g) can chickpeas, rinsed, drained

2 tsp finely grated lemon rind

1/3 cup fresh coriander leaves

Greek-style natural yoghurt, to serve

## Preparation

Heat oil in a saucepan over medium heat. Add onion and cook, stirring, for 5 minutes or until soft. Add the carrot, garlic, ginger, cumin seeds, paprika, cinnamon and saffron and cook, stirring, for 30 seconds or until aromatic.

Add stock and bring to the boil. Add the pumpkin, beans and apricots. Reduce heat to medium and cook, stirring occasionally, for 15 minutes or until the pumpkin is tender. Add dates, chickpeas and lemon rind and stir to combine.

Spoon among serving bowls and top with coriander. Serve with yoghurt.

## Thai Vegetable Curry

Serving 4
**List of Ingredients**
1 tablespoon peanut oil

17.60 oz (500g) sweet potato, peeled, cut into 3cm pieces

1 large brown onion, cut into thin wedges

2 garlic cloves, crushed

1/4 cup Ayam Thai red curry paste

400ml can coconut milk

1/2 cup chicken stock

1/2 quantity Roasted cauliflower with garlic (see related recipe)

8.80 oz (250g) snake beans, cut into 5cm lengths

10.60 oz (300g) silken firm tofu, cut into 3cm pieces

1 tablespoon fish sauce

1 tablespoon lime juice

1/2 cup chopped fresh coriander leaves

Steamed jasmine rice and lime wedges, to serve

## Preparation

Heat half the oil a large saucepan over medium-high heat. Add potato. Cook, stirring, for 5 minutes or until golden. Transfer to a plate.

Heat remaining oil in pan over medium heat. Add onion and garlic. Cook, stirring, for 3 minutes or until onion has softened. Add curry paste. Cook, stirring, for 1 minute or until fragrant.

Stir in coconut milk and stock. Bring to the boil. Add roasted cauliflower, beans and sweet potato. Reduce heat to low. Simmer, uncovered, for 10 to 12 minutes or until vegetables are tender. Add tofu, fish sauce, lime juice and half the coriander. Simmer for 2 minutes or until heated through. Divide rice between bowls. Spoon over curry and sprinkle with remaining coriander. Serve with lime wedges.

# Vegetarian Fried Brown Rice

Serving 4
**List of Ingredients**
2 eggs

2 teaspoons vegetable oil

1 onion, finely chopped

2 garlic cloves, crushed

1 red chili, finely chopped

1 large head broccoli, florets removed

1 large carrot, halved, thinly sliced

5.30 oz (150g) green beans, roughly chopped

2 cups brown basmati rice, cooked

2 tablespoons reduced-salt soy sauce or tamari

**Preparation**
Beat eggs with a fork until small bubbles appear. Heat a wok over medium-high heat until hot. Add 1 teaspoon of oil. Add eggs and swirl around wok to form a thin omelet. Cook for 1 minute. Turn and cook a further minute. Remove to a board. Thinly slice.

Add remaining oil, onion, garlic and chili to wok. Stir-fry for 2 minutes. Increase heat to high. Add broccoli, carrot and beans. Stir-fry for 4 minutes, or until tender and crisp.

Add rice and soy sauce or tamari to wok. Stir-fry for 3 minutes, or until heated through. Add egg and stir to combine. Serve immediately.

# Soup Recipes

## Hearty Sweet Potato Soup with Red Pepper

**List of Ingredients**
1 lb peeled cubed sweet potato
2 seeded and cubed red peppers
2 chopped cloves of garlic
1 chopped onion
10 ounces (300ml) dry white wine
41 ounces (1.2 L) chicken or vegetable stock (Light)
Salt and Pepper to taste
Bread to serve with soup

**Preparation**
Put the peeled cubed sweet potato, red peppers, garlic, onion, chicken/vegetable stock and wine into a saucepan and bring to the boil.
Allow to simmer for 30 min or until the vegetables are soft. Pour the mixture into a food processor or blender and blend until smooth and creamy. Serve warm with bread.

## Spinach and Green Pea Soup

**List of Ingredients**
1 cup finely sliced fresh spinach
1 chopped stick of celery
1.5 ounces finely chopped cabbage
½ finely shredded lettuce
2 1/2 cups frozen or fresh peas (podded)
2 crushed cloves of garlic
1 finely chopped leek
2 tbsp olive oil
1 tbsp finely chopped parsley
2/3 ounce (20 ml) shredded fresh mint
Salt and pepper to taste
41 ounces (1.2 L) chicken stock
2 slices of rindless back bacon
½ carton mustard and cress

**Preparation**
Place the leek, garlic, peas, bacon and stock in a large saucepan and bring to the boil. Allow to simmer for 20 min. When the first mixture is almost ready heat oil in a frying pan and add the lettuce, spinach, cabbage, herbs and celery. Cover and sweat over low heat until tender.
Now transfer the pea mixture into a blender and process until smooth.
Combine the blended mixture with the vegetables and herbs. Season with salt and pepper and serve with bread.

# Butternut Soup

**List of Ingredients**
1 large butternut squash
2 tbsp butter (unsalted)
1 chopped onion
Nutmeg to taste
6 cups chicken stock
Salt
Freshly ground black pepper

**Preparation**
Peel and seed the butternut and then cut into chunks.
Melt the butter in a large pot and fry the onions for a few minutes until they start to brown.
Add your chunks of butternut and the chicken stock and bring to a simmer.
Allow to simmer between 15 and 20 minutes or until the butternut is cooked through. It needs to be tender.
Remove the chunky pieces of squash and place them in a blender to make a puree.
Once blended place the squash back into the pot and finish off by seasoning with salt, pepper and nutmeg.

# Creamy Tomato Soup with a Peanut Surprise

**List of Ingredients**
1 tbsp olive oil
1 chopped onion
1 finely chopped green bell pepper
1 can crushed tomatoes
4 cups low-sodium chicken broth
¼ tsp Stevia powdered extract (2-3 drops Stevia liquid concentrate)
1 finely chopped celery stalk
1 chopped clove of garlic
1/2 tsp curry powder
1/2 tsp paprika
1/8 tsp cayenne pepper
Salt and black ground pepper to taste
1/3 cup peanut butter (preferably smooth)

**Preparation**
Heat the olive oil in a medium sized pan and fry the onions, peppers and celery for about 5 minutes. Now add the paprika, curry powder, garlic, 1 tsp salt and cayenne pepper and cook for a further 2 minutes.
Now add the chicken broth, Stevia, crushed tomatoes, and 1 cup of water. Using a whisk slowly add the peanut butter until properly blended.
Once the soup starts to boil, turn down the heat and simmer for a further 30 minutes stirring every now and then. The soup should have thickened by the time its ready.
Pour the soup into a blender and blend until a puree forms. Add salt and pepper to taste.

## Black Bean Vegetable Soup

Serving 8
**List of Ingredients**
1 1/2 cups (290g) dried black-eyed beans

4 cups (1L) cold water

4 cups (1L) vegetable stock

1 x 14.10 oz (400g) can diced tomatoes in juice

2 tbs tomato paste

1/4 tsp ground allspice

2 carrots, peeled, diced

2 celery sticks with leaves, diced

1 large brown onion, halved, finely chopped

1/4 cup loosely packed chopped fresh continental parsley leaves & stems

1 large garlic clove, crushed

Salt & freshly ground black pepper

1 tbs extra virgin olive oil

2 tbs chopped fresh continental parsley, extra, to garnish

**Preparation**

Place the beans in a bowl and cover with cold water. Set aside and soak overnight. Drain beans and rinse under cold water. Drain.

Combine water, stock, tomatoes, tomato paste and allspice in a large saucepan. Add the beans, carrot, celery, onion, parsley, garlic and bring to the boil over high heat. Reduce heat to low and cook, covered, for 1 1/2 hours or until beans are tender.

Taste and season with salt and pepper. Ladle into serving bowls. Drizzle with olive oil and sprinkle with the extra parsley to garnish. Serve immediately.

# Muesli, Nuts and Fruit Recipes

## Basic Muesli

Serving 8 cups
**List of Ingredients**
5 cups traditional rolled oats

1/2 cup processed bran

1/2 cup sunflower seeds

1/2 cup slivered almonds

1/2 cup sultanas

1/2 cup dried apricots, finely chopped

1/2 cup dried apple, finely chopped

Milk, fruit and honey, to serve

**Preparation**
Place oats, bran, sunflower seeds, almonds, sultanas, apricots and apple in an airtight container. Stir to combine.

Serve with milk, fruit and honey.

## Beans Almond Dukkah

Serving 4
**List of Ingredients**
3.50 oz (100g) Turkish bread, torn into 2cm pieces
17.60 oz (500g) green round beans, trimmed
2 tsp finely grated orange rind
2 tsp extra virgin olive oil
**Almond Dukkah**
1/3 cup (60g) blanched almonds
2 tbs sesame seeds
2 tsp ground coriander
2 tsp ground cumin
**Preparation**
Preheat oven to 392.00ºF (200ºC). Place the bread on a baking tray. Bake for 10 minutes or until light golden. Set aside to cool slightly. Break into small pieces.

Meanwhile, to make the almond dukkah, stir the almonds in a large frying pan over medium heat for 2-3 minutes or until lightly toasted. Transfer to a bowl. Cook sesame seeds in the pan, stirring, for 2 minutes or until lightly toasted. Add coriander and cumin. Cook, stirring, for 30 seconds or until aromatic. Transfer to a bowl. Finely chop the almonds. Stir into sesame mixture. Season with salt and pepper.

Cook the beans in a saucepan of salted boiling water for 2-3 minutes or until bright green and tender crisp. Drain.

Place bread, orange rind and 2 tablespoons of the dukkah in a bowl. Season with salt and pepper. Drizzle over the oil. Toss to combine.

Place the beans on a serving platter. Sprinkle with the bread mixture.

## Pecan Date Loaf

Serving 10
**List of Ingredients**
Melted reduced-fat dairy spread, to grease

7.10 oz (200g) fresh dates, pitted, coarsely chopped

1/3 cup (70g, firmly packed) brown sugar

1.80 oz (50g) reduced-fat dairy spread (Devondale Light brand)

1/2 cup (125ml) water

1 tsp bicarbonate of soda

1/2 cup (80g) whole meal plain flour

1 cup (160g) whole meal self-raising flour

1/2 tsp ground ginger

1/2 tsp ground cinnamon

1 egg, lightly whisked

1 tsp vanilla essence

1.80 oz (50g) pecans

## Preparation

Preheat oven to 356.00ºF (180°C). Brush a 9 x 19cm (base measurement) loaf pan with melted dairy spread to lightly grease. Line the base and sides with non-stick baking paper, allowing the 2 long sides to overhang.

Place the dates, sugar, dairy spread and water in a medium saucepan over medium heat. Cook, stirring, for 3 minutes or until the sugar dissolves. Add the bicarbonate of soda and stir until the mixture is well combined. Remove from heat and set aside, stirring occasionally, for 10 minutes or until mixture cools slightly.

Sift the combined flours, ginger and cinnamon into a large bowl. Return the husks to the flour mixture and make a well in the centre.

Add the egg and vanilla essence to the date mixture and use a fork to whisk until combined. Add the date mixture to j in the pecans. Spoon the mixture into the prepared pan and smooth the surface. Bake in preheated oven for 40 minutes or until a skewer inserted into the centre comes out clean. Remove the loaf from the oven and turn onto a wire rack to cool completely. Cut into slices to serve.

## Fig Bircher Muesli

Serving 4
**List of Ingredients**
2 1/2cups natural muesli

1 1/2 cups apple juice

1 cup reduced-fat plain yoghurt

3/4 cup reduced-fat milk

3/4 cup chopped dried figs

2 tablespoons honey

1/4 cup slivered almonds, toasted

3 fresh figs, quartered

**Preparation**
Combine muesli, apple juice, yoghurt, milk, dried figs and honey in a medium bowl. Cover and refrigerate overnight.

Spoon muesli mixture into bowls. Sprinkle with nuts. Top with fresh figs. Serve.

# Fruit Nut Mix

Serving 4
**List of Ingredients**
1/4 cup (45g) sultanas

1/4 cup (45g) whole blanched almonds

1.80 oz (50g) whole pitted dried dates

1/4 cup (35g) pecan halves

**Preparation**
Combine and mix all and keep in a small airtight container. Use as required. Keep in a cool cupboard for up to 1 month.

# Wholesome Homemade Berry Muesli

**List of Ingredients**
1 cup rolled oats
1/2 cup all-bran
1/4 cup dried cranberries
2 cups low-fat milk
1 sliced large banana
1/2 cup juicy fresh raspberries
**Preparation**
Mix the rolled oats, all bran and cranberries to make your muesli.

Place muesli in bowls and finish off by topping with raspberries, milk and banana slices. Guaranteed to be crispy and delicious!

# Honey Yoghurt Fruit Salad

Serving 4

**List of Ingredients**

8.80 oz (250g) strawberries, hulled, quartered

2 medium bananas, peeled, sliced

2 oranges, peeled, chopped

1 Fuji apple, chopped

7.10 oz (200g) light plain Greek-style yoghurt

1 tablespoon honey

1/3 cup almond kernels, chopped

**Preparation**

Combine strawberries, banana, orange and apple in a bowl.

Combine yoghurt and honey in a separate bowl.

Spoon fruit salad into bowls. Top with yoghurt mixture. Sprinkle with almonds. Serve.

## Oatsy Fruitsy Slices

Servings 16 pieces
**List of Ingredients**
5.30 oz (150g) dried apricots

3.50 oz (100g) dried apple

2 passionfruit, halved

2 tablespoons lemon juice

1/2 cup rolled oats

1/2 cup slivered almonds, toasted

1/4 cup pumpkin seeds (pepitas)

2 tablespoons linseed

**Topping**
- 2.60 oz (75g) dark chocolate, chopped
- 1/2 teaspoon olive oil

**Preparation**
Grease and line a 3cm-deep, 19cm x 29cm (base) slice pan with baking paper, allowing a 2cm overhang on both long ends.

Place apricots, apple, passionfruit pulp and lemon juice in a food processor. Process until just smooth. Transfer to a large bowl.

Process oats, almonds, pumpkin seeds and linseed until it resembles fine breadcrumbs. Add to fruit mixture. Stir to combine. Press mixture firmly into prepared pan. Refrigerate, covered for 1 hour or until slice is firm.

Line a tray with baking paper. Using a serrated knife, cut slice into 16 rectangular pieces. Place on prepared tray.

Make topping: Place chocolate and oil in a heatproof, microwave-safe bowl. Microwave on high (100%) for 1 1/2 to 2 minutes, stirring every 30 seconds with a metal spoon, or until melted and smooth. Spoon chocolate into a snap-lock bag. Snip off 1 corner and pipe chocolate over slice. Refrigerate until firm. Wrap in plastic wrap before packing into lunchboxes.

# Honeyed Macadamia Pears

Serving 4
**List of Ingredients**
4 firm ripe beurre bosc pears

1/3 cup honey

3/4 teaspoon ground cinnamon

1.10 oz (30g) unsalted roasted macadamia nuts, roughly chopped

2/3 cup natural low-fat yoghurt

**Preparation**
Cut pears lengthways into 1cm-thick slices. Heat honey and cinnamon in a large frying pan over low heat. Add pears. Cook for 2 to 3 minutes each side or until tender. Remove to a plate. Cover to keep warm.

Stir macadamia nuts into honey mixture. Cook, stirring, for 1 to 2 minutes or until syrup has reduced slightly.

Arrange pear slices on plates. Spoon over honeyed macadamia mixture. Serve with yoghurt.

# Orange Date Couscous

Serving 4
**List of Ingredients**
1 cup couscous

1 cup boiling water

1 large orange

1/2 cup pitted dried dates, halved

1 small carrot, peeled, grated

1 cup fresh mint leaves, finely chopped

1/4 cup pine nuts, toasted

1 tablespoon olive oil

1/2 teaspoon ground cumin

1 teaspoon caster sugar

**Preparation**
Place couscous in a heatproof bowl. Add boiling water. Cover. Set aside for 5 minutes or until liquid has absorbed. Using a fork, fluff to separate grains.

Meanwhile, peel and segment orange (see note). Squeeze membrane over a bowl to reserve juice (you'll need 1/4 cup). Discard membrane. Place couscous, orange segments, dates, carrot, mint and pine nuts in a bowl.

Place oil, cumin, sugar and reserved orange juice in a screw-top jar. Season with salt and pepper. Secure lid. Shake to combine. Pour over couscous mixture. Toss to combine. Serve.

## Orange Hummus

Serving 8

**List of Ingredients**

2 x 14.80 oz (420g) cans chickpeas, drained

1 1/2 tablespoons extra virgin olive oil

3 large oranges, rind finely grated, juiced

3 garlic cloves, crushed

1 tablespoon ground cumin

Pinch of cayenne pepper

2 tablespoons tahini

**Preparation**

Process chickpeas, oil, orange rind, 3/4 cup orange juice, garlic, cumin, cayenne pepper and tahini until smooth. Season with salt and pepper. Transfer to a bowl. Cover. Refrigerate until required.

# Roasted Cinnamon Pears

Serving 4
**List of Ingredients**
4 pears

Extra light olive oil spray

1 tablespoon caster sugar

1 teaspoon ground cinnamon

Low-fat ice-cream, to serve

Extra cinnamon, for sprinkling (optional)

**Preparation**
Preheat oven to 356.00°F (180°C). Peel pears and cut into quarters. Remove cores. Place in a large roasting pan lined with baking paper. Spray with oil.
Add combined sugar and cinnamon. Toss to coat. Roast for 20 minutes or until pears are tender and golden.
Serve roasted pears with low-fat ice-cream and sprinkle with extra cinnamon, if desired.

# Tropical Nut Mix

Serving 8

**List of Ingredients**

1 x 4.40 oz (125g) pkt pecan halves

1 x 4.40 oz (125g) pkt whole raw unsalted cashew nuts

1 x 3.50 oz (100g) pkt whole macadamia nuts

2 tsp olive oil

1/2 tsp ground cumin

1/2 tsp ground coriander

1/2 tsp garam marsala

1/4 tsp ground turmeric

Salt & freshly ground black pepper

1/2 cup (30g) flaked coconut

**Preparation**

Preheat oven to 356.00°F (180°C). Combine the pecans, cashews, macadamia nuts, oil, cumin, coriander, garam marsala and turmeric in a large bowl. Season with salt and pepper. Spread nut mixture evenly over a large baking tray. Roast in preheated oven, stirring occasionally, for 9 minutes or until nuts are toasted.

Add coconut and roast for a further 1 minute or until coconut is just toasted. Remove from oven and set aside for 30 minutes to cool before serving.

# Apples - Baked and Stuffed with Mixed Berries

**List of Ingredients**
4 apples
2 cups mixed berries (frozen)
4 cardamom pods
2 tsp honey
1/2 cup yoghurt

**Preparation**
Place the mixed berries in a sieve and put over a little bowl. Allow to that in the fridge overnight.
Preheat the oven to 320 deg. F (160 deg. Celsius).
Remove the cores from the 4 apples, forming a hole in each one that is 4cm in diameter.
Using a sharp knife, score around the entire circumference of each apple (aim for the center) and then make a small cut at the bottom where you will then insert a cardamom pod.
Divide 3/4 of the berries into the apples and before putting them into the over and baking for about 45 minutes, or until apples have softened considerably.
Place the rest of the berries in a little bowl and mash. Add the yoghurt and honey and stir.
Serve baked apples topped with yoghurt mixture.
Wholesome and delicious!

# Frozen Yoghurt filled with Mangoes, Berries, and Passion Fruit

**List of Ingredients**
1 medium sized mango
1 cup sliced strawberries
1/4 cup passion fruit pulp
2 cups vanilla yoghurt (low-fat)

**Preparation**
Place half of the berries and half of the mango into a blender separately and blend until smooth. Chop the remaining mango and berries and keep separate.

In a medium sized bowl combine 1/2 cup yoghurt, chopped mango and mango puree.

Divide this mixture amongst 8 X 8 ounce (250 ml) disposable cups and place in freezer for 1 hour. Remove once it has become firm.

Now combine 1/2 cup yoghurt, strawberry puree and remaining sliced strawberries. Distribute the strawberry amongst the 8 cups - on top of mango mixture. Place in freezer for 1 hour and remove once firm.

Combine the passion fruit pulp and remaining yoghurt. Divide the mixture between the 8 cups and place in freezer once again for an hour. Remove and push an ice cream stick into the centre of each cup.

Cover and freeze again for 3 hours. Remove when ready to serve.

# Frozen Bananas Smothered in Nuts

**List of Ingredients**
3 large ripe bananas
1/2 cup fat-free vanilla yogurt
½ cup Grape Nuts cereal

**Preparation**
Remove peels from bananas and cut each one in half (crosswise)

Push a wooden stick into the flat end of each banana and then spread vanilla yoghurt all over each one before rolling in the cereal.

Place bananas on wax paper and allow to freeze for about an hour. Serve frozen.

# Delicious Berry Salad

**List of Ingredients**
2 tbsp low-fat yoghurt
6 medium sized strawberries (remove stem and cut up)
¼ cup raspberries
¼ cup blueberries
1 tbsp lime juice
1 tbsp mint leaves
1 cup cantaloupe (cubed)

**Preparation**
Place all cut up fruit in a medium sized bowl.
Mix the lime juice, yoghurt, and mint together and then add to the fruit and toss. Serve chilled.

# Berry Peach and Apple Salad

**List of Ingredients**
1 cup raspberries
1 cup blackberries
1 cup strawberries
1 sliced apples
1 sliced peach
2 cups chopped lettuce
1 tsp crushed almonds
**Preparation**
Place all ingredients in a large bowl and toss for a refreshing and healthy snack.

# Very Berry Popsicle

**List of Ingredients**
1 cup black cherries
1 cup blackberries
1 cup water
1/2 tsp ginger
1 cup fat free berry yoghurt
1 cup orange juice (100%, unsweetened)
**Preparation**
Place all the ingredients in a blender and strain before placing in a popsicle tray and freezing.

# Icy Banana and Berry Delight

**List of Ingredients**
1 cup strawberries
1 cup blueberries
1/2 banana peeled and sliced
1/2 tsp ginger
1 cup water
1 cup roughly chopped pineapple

**Preparation**
Place fruit in medium sized bowl and sprinkle ginger over. Toss and then add water. Place ingredients in your popsicle tray and freeze for a chunky icy surprise.

# Smoothie Recipes

# Refreshing Peach Smoothie

**List of Ingredients**
2 cups peach slices
1 cup fat-free peach yogurt with no-calorie sweetener
1cup crushed ice or ice cubes
**Preparation**
Blend with a blender until smooth.

# Blueberry Peach Smoothie

**List of Ingredients**
2 cups peach slices
½ cup blueberries
1 cup fat free vanilla yoghurt
1 cup crushed ice or ice cubes
**Preparation**
Blend with a blender until smooth.

# Strawberry and Peach Smoothie

**List of Ingredients**
2 cups peach slices
½ cup strawberries
1 cup fat free strawberry yoghurt
1 cup crushed ice or ice cubes
**Preparation**
Blend with a blender until smooth.

## Banana Strawberry Smoothie

**List of Ingredients**
2 cups diced strawberries
1sliced medium banana
1 cup fat free vanilla yoghurt
1cup ice cubes or crushed ice
1sliced kiwi fruit for garnish

**Preparation**
In a blender combine all the fruit and yoghurt and blend.
Slowly add the ice cubes and continue blending until smooth.

## Coffee Vanilla Smoothie

**List of Ingredients**
1 cup low fat vanilla yogurt
1/3 cup fat free milk
½ cup ice cubes/crushed ice
1 tsp instant coffee
**Preparation**
Blend with a blender until smooth.

# Strawberry Honey Twist Smoothie

**List of Ingredients**
½ medium sized banana, sliced
½ cup fresh strawberries
1 tsp ginger
1/4 cup dry milk powder (non-fat)
1/4 cup apple juice
1 tbsp honey
1 cup ice cubes/crushed ice
**Preparation**
Blend with a blender until smooth.

# Almond Blueberry Smoothie

**List of Ingredients**
1.5 cups fresh blueberries
1/2 cup fat free Greek yoghurt
2 tbsp wheat germ
2 tbsp skim milk
1/4 cup almonds
2 tsp honey
1 cup ice cubes/crushed ice
**Preparation**
Blend with a blender until smooth.

# Raspberry Peanut Surprise Smoothie

**List of Ingredients**
1.5 cups fresh raspberries
2 tbsp skim milk
2 tsp honey
2 tbsp smooth peanut butter
1 cup ice cubes
**Preparation**
Blend with a blender until smooth.

# Spinach Apple Smoothie

**List of Ingredients**
1 medium sized apple, sliced
2 cups spinach
1/2 cup fat-free Greek Yoghurt
1/3 cup pure apple juice
2 tbsp flax seeds
1 cup ice cubes/crushed ice
1 tsp honey
**Preparation**
Blend with a blender until smooth.

# Cottage Cheese, Raspberry and Cinnamon Smoothie

**List of Ingredients**
1.5 cups raspberries
1/2 cup fat free cottage cheese
1 tsp honey
Pinch of cinnamon
2 tbsp rolled oats
1 cup ice cubes/crushed ice
**Preparation**
Blend with a blender until smooth.

## Blackberry and Honey Smoothie

**List of Ingredients**
1.5 cups fresh blackberries
1/2 cup plain fat-free Greek yogurt
2 tsp honey
2 tablespoons almond butter
1 cup ice cubes
**Preparation**
Blend with a blender until smooth.

## Berry and Banana Smoothie

**List of Ingredients**
2 cups plain non-fat yogurt
2 bananas, sliced
1 cup fresh strawberries, sliced
1 cup fresh raspberries (alternatively use blueberries or blackberries)
**Preparation**
Blend with a blender until smooth.

# Pineapple and Coconut Smoothie

**List of Ingredients**
1 cup fat free or low- fat plain yogurt
1.5 cups fresh pineapple, sliced
1 tsp coconut extract (non-alcoholic)
1 cup ice cubes/crushed ice
**Preparation**
Blend with a blender until smooth.

## Banana and Green Tea Smoothie

**List of Ingredients**
1 medium sized banana, sliced
1 cup skim milk
3 tbsp hot water
2 tsps green tea powder
1 cup crushed ice/ ice cubes

**Preparation**
First combine the green tea powder and hot water to form a paste.
Place all the other ingredients, including the paste into a blender and blend until smooth.

## Breakfast Smoothie

**List of Ingredients**
1/2 cup dry oats (uncooked)
1 1/2 cups skim milk
1 small banana, sliced
1 tbsp flaxseed
1 tsp coffee extract
**Preparation**
Place oats in blender and blend until they become powdery. Add the rest of the ingredients and blend until smooth.

# Caramel Peanut Smoothie

**List of Ingredients**
1 cup unsweetened almond milk
1/2 cup skim milk
2 pkts Splenda
1 tbsp unsweetened cocoa powder
1 tbsp peanut butter
1 tbsp sugar free caramel syrup
1 tbsp ground flax seed
3/4 scoop protein powder (Preferably Vanilla)
**Preparation**
Place all ingredients in blender and blend until smooth

# Strawberry and Cinnamon Smoothie

**List of Ingredients**
1 cup fresh strawberries
1/2 cup fat-free vanilla yoghurt
1/2 cup skim milk
3 tbsp flax meal
1/2 tsp cinnamon
**Preparation**
Blend with a blender until smooth.

### Banana Mango Smoothie

**List of Ingredients**
1 large mango, peeled and sliced
2 medium sized bananas, sliced
2 cup orange juice
2 tbsp maple syrup
1/2 cup plain fat free yogurt
1/8 tsp ground cardamom

**Preparation**
Place all ingredients except maple syrup into blender and blend until smooth.
Slowly add maple syrup to taste.

# Bibliography

1. Encyclopedia of Natural Medicine Revised 2nd Edition: Michael Murray N.D. and Joseph Pizzorno N.D.
2. Alternative Medicine: The Definitive Guide; Second Edition: Larry Trivieri, JR Editor, Introduced by Burton Goldberg.
3. Alternative Cures: Bill Gottlieb
4. "The Great Cholesterol Lie: Why Inflammation Kills and the Real Cure for Heart Disease" Dr. Dwight Lundell

# More Books by John McArthur

**Hypothyroidism**

**Hypothyroidism: The Hypothyroidism Solution.** Hypothyroidism Natural Treatment and Hypothyroidism Diet for Under Active Or Slow Thyroid, Causing Weight Loss Problems, Fatigue, Cardiovascular Disease. John McArthur (Author), Cheri Merz (Editor)

## Fibromyalgia And Chronic Fatigue

**Fibromyalgia And Chronic Fatigue:** A Step-By-Step Guide For Fibromyalgia Treatment And Chronic Fatigue Syndrome Treatment. Includes Fibromyalgia Diet And Chronic Fatigue Diet And Lifestyle Guidelines. John McArthur (Author), Cheri Merz (Editor)

## Yeast Infection

**Candida Albicans:** Yeast Infection Treatment. Treat Yeast Infections With This Home Remedy. The Yeast Infection Cure. John McArthur (Author)

## Heart Disease

**Hypertension - High Blood Pressure:** How To Lower Blood Pressure Permanently In 8 Weeks Or Less, The Hypertension Treatment, Diet and Solution. John McArthur (Author)

**Cholesterol Myth:** Lower Cholesterol Won't Stop Heart Disease. Healthy Cholesterol Will. Cholesterol Recipe Book & Cholesterol Diet. Lower Cholesterol Naturally Keep Cholesterol Healthy. John McArthur (Author), Cheri Merz (Editor)

**Heart Disease Prevention and Reversal:** How To Prevent, Cure and Reverse Heart Disease Naturally For A Healthy Heart. John McArthur (Author)

## Diabetes

**Diabetes Diet:** Diabetes Management Options. Includes a Diabetes Diet Plan with Diabetic Meals and Natural Diabetes Food, Herbs and Supplements for Total Diabetes Control. Delicious Recipes. John McArthur (Author), Corinne Watson (Editor)

**Diabetes Cooking:** 93 Diabetes Recipes for Breakfast, Lunch, Dinner, Snacks and Smoothies. A Guide to Diabetes Foods to Help You Prepare Healthy Delicious ... Diabetic Meals and Natural Diabetes Food) John McArthur (Author), Corinne Watson (Editor)

## Stress and Anxiety

**From Stressful to Successful in 4 Easy Steps:** Stress at Work? Stress in Relationship? Be Stress Free. End Stress and Anxiety. Excellent Stress Management, Stress Control and Stress Relief Techniques. John McArthur (Author)

**Anxiety and Panic Attacks:** Anxiety Management. Anxiety Relief. The Natural And Drug Free Relief For Anxiety Attacks, Panic Attacks And Panic Disorder. John McArthur (Author), Cheri Merz (Editor)

## Back and Neck Pain

**The 15 Minute Back Pain and Neck Pain Management Program:** Back Pain and Neck Pain Treatment and Relief 15 Minutes a Day No Surgery No Drugs. Effective, Quick and Lasting Back and Neck Pain Relief. John McArthur (Author)

## Arthritis

**Arthritis:** Arthritis Relief for Osteoarthritis, Rheumatoid Arthritis, Gout, Psoriatic Arthritis, and Juvenile Arthritis. Follow The Arthritis Diet, Cure and Treatment Free Yourself From The Pain. John McArthur (Author)

## Depression

**How to Break the Grip of Depression:** Read How Robert Declared War On Depression ... And Beat It! John McArthur (Author)

## Pregnancy

**Pregnancy Nutrition:** Pregnancy Food. Pregnancy Recipes. Healthy Pregnancy Diet. Pregnancy Health. Pregnancy Eating and Recipes. Nutritional Tips and 63 Delicious Recipes for Moms-to-Be. Corinne Watson (Author), John McArthur (Author)

**Pregnancy and Childbirth:** Expecting a Baby. Pregnancy Guide. Pregnancy What to Expect. Pregnancy Health. Pregnancy Eating and Recipes. Cheri Merz (Author), John McArthur (Author)

## Allergies
**Allergy Free:** Fast Effective Drug-free Relief for Allergies. Allergy Diet. Allergy Treatments. Allergy Remedies. Natural Allergy Relief. John McArthur (Author), Cheri Merz (Editor)

Printed in Great Britain
by Amazon